◌ **Collins** *gem*

Calorie Counter

D0558732

This book has been compiled with the assistance of hundreds of brand-name manufacturers. Other sources are listed on page 48.

HarperCollins Publishers
Westerhill Road, Bishopbriggs, Glasgow G64 2QT

www.collins.co.uk

First published 1984
Eighth edition published 2006

Reprint 10 9 8 7 6 5 4 3 2 1

© HarperCollins Publishers 2006

ISBN 0 00 721150 3

Typeset by Davidson Pre-Press Graphics Ltd, Glasgow

Printed in Italy by Amadeus Srl

PREFACE

The *Collins Gem Calorie Counter* is one of the most successful guides available for weight watchers. In this new edition, we give a new selection of foods, reflecting the range of foods now available in our shops and have updated all the nutritional data. The book contains:

- An introduction that explains about weight loss, the targets you may need to set, and how to live with a Calorie-controlled diet.
- A listing of around 6,000 foods, including both everyday ingredients and thousands of branded foods available in shops today. The entries are organised in sections reflecting shop arrangements. Study the Contents pages (pages 5–8) and the Index to help identify the foods you are looking for.
- Two separate listings for Kid's Foods and for Fast Foods are also given.
- For each entry we give information on the following: Calories, protein, carbohydrates, fat and fibre.

It has long been known that the healthiest and most effective way to lose weight is to combine a Calorie controlled diet with exercise. We hope that this guide will help you plan the best way to restrict your Calorie intake.

USEFUL WEBSITES

www.caloriecontrol.org/bmi (*easy-to-use imperial BMI calculator and waist circumference chart*)

www.nhlbisupport.com/bmi (*metric and imperial BMI calculator*)

www.caloriescount.com (*advice about healthy eating and fitness on a Calorie-controlled diet*)

www.healthyweightforum.org (*support, motivation, recipes and fellowship for slimmers*)

www.fdf.org.uk (*healthy lifestyle initiative combining healthy eating and fitness tips*)

www.weightconcern.com (*addresses physical and psychological needs of overweight people*)

www.bbc.co.uk/health/healthy_living/your_weight/ (*excellent site with medical advice, tips, eating well, fitness and useful contacts*)

www.nutrition.org.uk (*good, sensible advice based on research; can put you in touch with a nutritionist.*)

www.weightlossresources.co.uk (*wide range of information on boosting metabolism, burning Calories and exercise*)

www.stayinginshape.com (*handy calculator to work out number of Calories burned*)

www.bupa.co.uk/health_information (*resources for losing weight the healthy way, with fun quizzes*)

www.recipezaar.com (*low-Calorie recipes from around the world*)

CONTENTS

INTRODUCTION

The main diet news story of the 21st century so far has been about limiting the quantities and types of carbohydrate foods you eat. Plans like Atkins and the South Beach Diet advocate high-protein and very low-carb meals, while the GI and GL diets advise that you opt for carbs that are slowly metabolised so don't have a dramatic impact on your blood sugar levels. Do they work? It's true that the glycaemic index (GI) can be a valuable tool to prevent cravings and hunger pangs while you lose weight, but it provides nothing like the full story. Meanwhile, Atkins Nutritionals has filed for bankruptcy in the US. The bottom line is that there is no magic solution. No diets will work if you continue to consume too many Calories, even if they come from 'permitted foods'. Put simply, it's Calories – not carbs – that make you gain weight.

If you want to lose weight, the basic truth is that you have to burn off more energy (measured in kilocalories, often shortened to Calories, with a capital C) than you take in through food. To make sure you do this reasonably accurately, you will have to count the Calories in the food you eat and liquids you drink. This doesn't mean that you have to walk around for the rest of your life with this book in one hand and a calculator in the other. Successful dieters become 'Calorie aware' and able to spot the low-Calorie, nutritionally sound option at a glance. This book will help you to learn the values for all your favourites and serve as a quick reference in which to look up new foods.

Before you start, you need to find out how many Calories you burn per day, then calculate how many you can get away with eating when trying to lose (or maintain) weight.

HOW ARE CALORIES BURNED OFF?

Energy is burned in three ways. The most important of these is your Resting Metabolic Rate (RMR), which accounts for between 65 and 75 per cent of all the energy you burn. RMR is the amount of energy your body expends while at rest, on processes like heartbeat, circulation, breathing, the release of hormones, and maintaining your body temperature. RMR varies from person to person, partly because muscle burns more energy than fat, even when you're not moving. A kilogram of muscle can burn more than 120 kilocalories a day at rest, while a kilogram of fat burns 20 kcal or less. So the more muscle you have, the higher your RMR is likely to be, and the more energy you will burn without trying.

The second way to burn energy is known as the Thermic Effect of Food, and it represents the amount of energy required to digest food. It's generally around 10 per cent of the Calories eaten, so digesting a 500-Calorie lunch could burn off 50 Calories.

FAD DIETS

Avoid any diets that suggest you omit an entire food group or eat a so-called 'miracle food'. Steer clear of any that promise rapid weight loss or that don't recommend you exercise as well as curtailing your eating. A realistic weight loss is between 5 and 10 per cent of your body weight over six months. Any more than this and you will struggle to keep it off.

The third way to burn energy is the Thermic Effect of Exercise. The chart on pages 14-15 gives some average values for the amount of energy you might burn during different types of exercise, depending on your body weight. These might not be as high as you'd expect; for example, a 60 kg woman jogging for half an hour would only burn 245 kcal and a 75 kg man cycling for half an hour would burn 240 kcal.

The most effective way to burn more Calories is to raise your Resting Metabolic Rate by developing a more active lifestyle and forming more muscle while shrinking your fat deposits. The International Association for the Study of Obesity recommends that we all get 60 minutes of moderate-intensity exercise a day, and research shows that this is most effective when broken up into smaller chunks throughout the day. If you walk or cycle to work, always take the stairs rather than the elevator, and do some energetic housework or gardening when you get home, you could easily make up the 60 minutes total without setting foot in a gym.

On the other hand, if you diet too drastically, cutting your Calorie intake below 1500 day, your Resting Metabolic Rate could decrease as your body goes into starvation mode and takes steps to protect itself. The bad news is that your RMR will also decrease as you get older, by roughly 2 per cent for each decade over the age of 20, unless you take very positive steps to keep it high. And genetics comes into it. If you had an overweight parent, you are 79 per cent more likely to struggle with your own weight (this percentage is even higher if it was your mum).

HOW MANY CALORIES CAN YOU EAT?

Here's a quick formula for calculating roughly how many Calories you can consume in a day without gaining weight:

- If you are a woman with a largely sedentary lifestyle (desk job, car, little time to exercise), multiply your weight in kilos by 26 to get the number of Calories you should eat a day to maintain your current weight.
- If you are a sedentary man, multiply your weight in kg by 31.
- If you are an active woman (getting 60 minutes of moderate-intensity exercise a day plus three sessions of aerobic exercise a week), multiply your weight in kg by 33.
- If you are an active man, multiply your weight in kg by 37.
- If you are a very active woman (getting 60 minutes of moderate-intensity exercise a day plus five to seven sessions of aerobic exercise a week), multiply your weight in kg by 39.
- If you are a very active man, multiply your weight in kg by 44.

It has been calculated that a kilogram of weight is equivalent to 7,700 Calories, so for every kilo a dieter wants to lose, 7,700 Calories must be cut from the diet or burned through exercise (or preferably both). Sensible weight loss to aim at is around 0.5 kg a week, and to achieve this you would have to consume 3,350 Calories fewer a week – or 478 fewer a day.

Number of Calories burned in
30 minutes of activity (in relation to body weight)

Activity/exercise	50kg	55kg	60kg	65kg	70kg	75kg
Aerobics	155	170	185	200	225	250
Badminton	190	200	210	220	230	240
Basketball	310	350	390	430	470	500
Bowling	95	100	105	110	115	120
Canoeing	120	125	135	140	145	150
Carpentry	125	135	140	145	150	160
Cooking	70	75	80	85	90	95
Cycling	150	165	180	195	210	240
Dancing, moderate	115	120	130	135	140	150
Dancing, fast	300	310	320	330	340	350
Dish-washing	70	75	80	85	90	95
Driving	50	55	60	65	70	75
Exercise, moderate	150	160	170	180	190	200
Exercise, fast	200	220	240	260	280	300
Football	275	300	325	350	375	400
Gardening	120	130	140	150	160	170
Golf, no cart	120	125	130	140	145	150
Golf, with cart	70	75	80	85	90	95
Handball	260	275	290	310	330	350
Hockey (field or ice)	300	310	320	330	340	350
Horseback-riding	130	140	150	160	170	180
Housework, active	100	105	110	120	125	135

Activity/exercise	50kg	55kg	60kg	65kg	70kg	75kg
Ironing	70	70	75	75	80	80
Jogging, light	225	235	245	255	265	275
Lacrosse	300	315	330	345	360	375
Office work	65	70	75	80	85	90
Painting (walls)	130	135	140	150	160	170
Piano playing	100	105	110	115	120	125
Reading	15	15	20	20	25	25
Rowing	325	350	375	400	425	450
Running, slow	290	315	345	375	405	435
Running, fast	375	415	450	490	525	550
Sewing	25	25	30	30	35	35
Singing	35	40	45	50	55	60
Sitting at rest	15	15	20	20	25	25
Skating, energetically	250	260	270	280	290	300
Skiing, energetically	250	260	270	280	290	300
Stair climbing	170	185	200	215	230	250
Sweeping floor	70	75	80	90	100	110
Swimming, slow	190	210	230	250	270	290
Swimming, fast	240	260	285	305	330	355
Tennis	165	180	195	215	230	245
Typing	85	90	95	100	105	110
Volleyball	170	185	200	215	230	250
Walking, moderately	105	115	125	135	145	155
Walking, fast	125	135	145	155	165	175

In fact, this would be quite realistic for most people – but you shouldn't go lower than 1,500 Calories a day except under medical supervision.

- If you've got 20 kg to lose, allow yourself up to 40 weeks.
- If you've got 15 kg to lose, allow up to 30 weeks.
- If you've got 10 kg to lose, allow up to 20 weeks.
- If you've got 5 kg to lose, allow up to 10 weeks.
- And you should be able to lose 2 kg in 4 weeks, and 1 kg in 2 weeks.

Trying to lose weight more quickly than this is counter-productive, as crash diets can have all sorts of unwanted side effects, including the following.

- Your metabolism will slow down as your body tries to protect its fat stores, making it more difficult to shed weight. Once you stop dieting, this low metabolism will remain, and you are likely to pile the weight back on again.
- You will burn up muscle tissue rather than fat. Muscle tissue burns more Calories than fat tissue, so your rate of weight loss could slow down.
- Deprivation dieting or skipping meals can cause a drop in blood sugar levels, which leads to sugar cravings and an urge to binge.
- The more extreme your diet, the greater the likelihood that you will not be able to stick to it.

WARNING

Anyone who is considering trying to lose a lot of weight should consult their doctor first. You should also talk to your doctor before starting a diet if you have any long-term health problems or take medication for chronic conditions like diabetes, angina, epilepsy or osteoporosis.

You should start to lose weight soon after you cut down the number of Calories you consume, but in the long term you'll get ill if you don't ensure that you eat a balanced diet with all the recommended nutrients. The *Calorie Counter* doesn't just list the Calorie content of each food, but also gives the nutritional composition. On pages 29-41 there is an explanation of the elements required in a healthy diet.

If you keep dieting and exercising without achieving your target, it may be that you are being unrealistic and trying to reach a weight that is unhealthy for your height, body frame and metabolism. Here's how to calculate the ideal weight for your body shape.

FINDING YOUR IDEAL WEIGHT

Everyone is born with a 'natural weight range', at which they feel healthiest and most attractive. It might vary naturally throughout the year – some put on a little more weight in winter and shed it in summer, while women can gain as much as 2 kg around their periods due to water retention. It can also tend to increase with age as your Resting Metabolic Rate slows down.

If you consistently eat too much and don't exercise, it is possible to reach a weight well above this natural range. It is much harder to maintain a weight that is below your natural range. Long-term dieters, especially 'crash dieters', can end up confusing their metabolism, so that they gain weight quickly as soon as they stop dieting.

Charts that give ideal weight ranges for your height, such as the one on pages 20-21, are just approximations that reflect cultural averages. Two people of the same height can have completely different weights and yet both be healthy. Muscle weighs more than fat, so someone who exercises regularly might weigh more than someone of the same height who is sedentary. Weight also depends on body frame, so you should calculate whether you are small, medium or large-framed before consulting height and weight charts.

The easiest way to do this is to measure around the narrowest part of your wrist and then check the list below to see if you have a small, medium or large frame. (If you don't know your height in metres, see the conversion chart on page 49.)

Women
Height under 1.58 m:
- Small frame = wrist size less than 14 cm
- Medium frame = wrist size 14 cm to 15 cm
- Large frame = wrist size over 15 cm
Height 1.58 to 1.65 m:
- Small frame = wrist size less than 15 cm
- Medium frame = wrist size 15 cm to 16 cm
- Large frame = wrist size over 16 cm
Height over 1.65 m:
- Small frame = wrist size less than 16 cm
- Medium frame = wrist size 16 cm to 17 cm
- Large frame = wrist size over 17 cm

Men
Height under 1.65 m:
- Small frame = wrist size less than 16 cm
- Medium frame = wrist size 16 cm to 17 cm
- Large frame = wrist size over 17 cm
Height over 1.65 m:
- Small frame = wrist size less than 17 cm
- Medium frame = wrist size 17 cm to 19 cm
- Large frame = wrist size over 19 cm

Tables for Standard Body Weight

Men

Height m (ft)	Small Frame kg (lbs)	Medium Frame kg (lbs)	Large Frame kg (lbs)
1.55 (5'1")	49–59 (107–130)	51–61 (113–134)	55–64 (121–140)
1.57 (5'2")	50–60 (110–132)	53–63 (116–138)	56–65 (124–144)
1.60 (5'3")	51–61 (113–134)	54–64 (119–140)	58–68 (127–150)
1.63 (5'4")	53–61 (116–135)	55–65 (122–142)	59–70 (131–154)
1.65 (5'5")	54–62 (119–137)	57–66 (125–146)	60–72 (133–159)
1.68 (5'6")	56–64 (122–140)	59–68 (129–149)	62–74 (137–163)
1.70 (5'7")	58–65 (127–143)	60–69 (133–152)	64–76 (142–167)
1.73 (5'8")	60–66 (131–145)	62–71 (137–155)	66–78 (146–171)
1.75 (5'9")	61–68 (135–149)	64–72 (141–158)	68–80 (150–175)
1.78 (5'10")	63–69 (139–152)	66–73 (145–161)	70–81 (154–179)
1.80 (5'11")	65–70 (143–155)	68–75 (149–165)	72–83 (159–183)
1.83 (6')	67–72 (147–159)	70–77 (153–169)	74–85 (163–187)
1.85 (6'1")	69–75 (151–165)	71–80 (157–175)	76–86 (167–189)
1.88 (6'2")	70–76 (155–168)	73–81 (161–179)	78–89 (171–197)
1.90 (6'3")	72–79 (157–173)	75–84 (166–185)	80–92 (176–202)

Women

Height m (ft)	Small Frame kg (lbs)	Medium Frame kg (lbs)	Large Frame kg (lbs)
1.47 (4'10")	41–49 (91–108)	43–52 (95–115)	47–54 (103–119)
1.50 (4'11")	42–51 (93–112)	44–55 (98–121)	48–57 (106–125)
1.52 (5')	44–52 (96–115)	46–57 (101–124)	49–58 (109–128)
1.55 (5'1")	45–54 (99–118)	47–58 (104–127)	51–59 (112–131)
1.57 (5'2")	46–55 (102–121)	49–60 (107–132)	52–61 (115–135)
1.60 (5'3")	48–56 (105–124)	50–62 (110–135)	54–63 (118–138)
1.63 (5'4")	49–58 (108–127)	51–63 (113–138)	55–65 (122–142)
1.65 (5'5")	50–59 (111–130)	53–64 (117–141)	57–66 (126–145)
1.68 (5'6")	52–60 (115–133)	55–66 (121–144)	59–67 (130–148)
1.70 (5'7")	54–62 (119–136)	57–67 (125–147)	61–69 (134–151)
1.73 (5'8")	56–63 (123–139)	58–68 (128–150)	62–71 (137–155)
1.75 (5'9")	58–64 (127–142)	60–69 (133–153)	64–73 (141–159)
1.78 (5'10")	59–66 (131–145)	62–71 (137–156)	66–75 (146–165)
1.80 (5'11")	61–68 (135–148)	64–72 (141–159)	68–77 (150–170)
1.83 (6')	63–69 (138–151)	65–74 (143–163)	69–79 (153–173)

Body Mass Index

Doctors and health professionals are likely to use the Body Mass Index (BMI) – a height to weight formula – to calculate whether you are over- or underweight. To find your BMI, divide your weight in kilograms by the square of your height in metres, i.e. weight ÷ height^2. Check your total against the list below to see if you fall into an average range.

For example, if you are 1.75 m tall and weigh 64 kg,
1.75 x 1.75 = 3.06
64 ÷ 3.06 = 20.91

BMI scale:

less than 15	emaciated
15–18.9	underweight
19–24.9	average
25–29.9	overweight
30+	obese

If your BMI is in the emaciated or obese range in this scale, you should visit your doctor for advice as you could be seriously endangering your health.

You can use the BMI to establish a healthy weight that you want to achieve. For example, let's say you are 1.83 metres tall and weigh 95 kg, so you have a

BMI of $95 \div 3.35 = 28.36$. This puts you in the overweight category. Say you want to reduce your BMI to 24, you multiply your height squared by 24:

$$(1.83 \times 1.83) \times 24 = 80.4$$

This is the weight you should slim down to to get back in the healthy range, so you have $95 - 80.4 = 14.6$ kg to lose. Referring back to page 16, you'll see that this should take you up to 30 weeks.

BMI is a useful tool, although it doesn't give any indication of where fat is stored in the body, which will affect the health risks you face, and there are several groups for whom the formula doesn't apply. Heavily muscled athletes or pregnant women could appear overweight on the BMI scale while being perfectly healthy. There are different BMI scales for children and adolescents (see pages 26-29) and some ethnic groups have different BMI ratings as well; for example, the World Health Organisation states that a BMI of 27.5 for an Asian carries the same health risks as a BMI of 30 for a Caucasian.

Even if it's obvious where you are carrying excess weight, it is worth checking your waist measurement as well as your BMI to get the whole picture.

Waist circumference

Those who carry a lot of excess fat round the waist are in the highest-risk category for high blood pressure, heart disease and strokes – this country's biggest killers. If your waist measurement rises above 102 cm (40 inches) for men and above 88 cm (35 inches) for women, you are putting yourself at serious risk and should start a weight-loss programme with plenty of fat-burning aerobic exercise as soon as possible.

Another measure that indicates those at high risk is the waist-to-hip ratio (WHR). The waist is measured at the narrowest point and that figure is divided by the hip measurement at the widest point. A high WHR is more than 1.0 in men and above 0.85 in women. A healthy value is anything below these.

KEEPING IT OFF

A study by the National Weight Control Registry in the US follows a group of dieters who have lost at least 14 kg each and kept it off for a year or more. The secrets of their success are that they all eat a low-fat, high-carb diet, they weigh themselves regularly so they can see if the kilos are starting to pile back on, and they each get between 60 and 90 minutes of moderate-intensity exercise a day.

Research suggests that long-term chronic stress can cause us to lay down more fat round our waistlines, and excessive consumption of alcohol can have the same effect. Take steps to deal with your stress, and control your drinking, and you could see the benefits on your figure – and your overall health – before too long.

Charting your diet progress

Weighing yourself every single morning could be confidence-destroying, because there will be days when you have put on a pound despite your best efforts, and others when your weight doesn't seem to shift at all. When you start a weight-loss diet, use the BMI scale to work out your target healthy weight and take a set of starting measurements – such as chest, waist, hips, thighs and upper arms. Thereafter weigh yourself just once a week (at the same time of day, and either naked or wearing the same clothes). Note your weight in a notebook or on a chart. Once a month, take your measurements again, so you can see where you are losing the weight from. If you want to lose from your hips and it's only shifting from your chest, look into exercises that specifically target the hips (a gym instructor should be able to help).

It is also a good idea to keep a food diary when you are dieting. Write down everything you eat at the time and work out your subtotals as you go along, so you can see whether you can afford that glass of wine in the evening or not. Don't try to remember later what you have eaten, as you will inevitably forget some items and misremember portion size!

Tot up your daily Calorie intake and compare it with the chart on which you note your weight loss. You should be able to see the correlation. Keeping account of your Calorie intake is a helpful strategy for staying on track – especially once you can see that you lose less weight in weeks when you exceed your Calorie allowance. It's not an exact science, because other factors come into play, but no one has yet come up with a more reliable way of losing weight and keeping it off long-term than cutting back your Calorie intake to less than the number you burn.

CHILDREN'S WEIGHT

Paediatricians and other health professionals are becoming increasingly concerned about the rising rates of obesity in British children. According to statistics, 17 per cent of children in the West are currently obese (that's not just overweight, but seriously endangering their health). If the trend continues, it's predicted that by 2020, one in five boys and one in three girls will be obese. And it's not just

GETTING HELP

If you are concerned about your child's weight, talk to your GP first of all. Weight Concern (tel. 020 7679 6636; www.weightconcern.com) and the Institute of Child Health (020 7242 9789; www.ich.ucl.ac.uk) are useful sources of advice, and the book *How to Help Your Overweight Child*, by Karen Sullivan, is well worth reading for its practical suggestions.

'puppy fat' that they'll 'grow out of'. Forty per cent of obese seven-year-olds and seventy per cent of obese adolescents will become obese adults.

So how can you tell if your child is overweight? The BMI scale for adults doesn't apply to children, because it is natural for their weight-to-height ratio to vary at different stages. Very young children have more baby fat, but once they become more active their BMI declines until the age of about five or six, then increases through to adolescence. The government now supplies paediatric BMI charts in health booklets and you will be able to track your child's height and weight according to their 'percentile band'.

There are nine percentile lines: 99.6th, 98th, 91st, 75th, 50th, 25th, 9th, 2nd and 0.4th. These are just a measure of how your child's scores compare with the average, which is the 50th percentile line. Children above the 50th line are bigger than average for their age and children below this are smaller, but high or low readings don't necessarily indicate a problem. Doctors look for steady growth; your child should stay more or less on the same line as he or she grows.

- If your child's height falls above the 99.6th or below the 0.4th percentile line, you will probably be referred to a paediatrician who can test for growth hormone problems.
- For a child aged under five, if their weight goes up or down by the width of one whole percentile band (the distance between two percentile lines) in the course of a year or 18 months, you should consult a doctor. If it goes up or down by two-thirds of a band, keep an eye on it and re-assess the following year.
- For children over five, if their weight veers up or down by two-thirds of a percentile band in the course of 12 to 18 months, you should see a doctor. If it veers by half a band, re-measure in 12 months.

The important thing is not to panic and put your child on a diet if you think they are overweight. The single most important thing you can teach them is to be active people, by playing sports, cycling, swimming and, whenever possible, getting outside to run around instead of sitting in front of the TV. Experts recommend that children get 60 minutes of at least moderate-intensity exercise every day – but currently two in ten get less than 30 minutes.

When choosing food for your children, read the labels carefully. Some foods designed for kids have horrifying levels of fat, sugar and salt. Choose products with less than 10 g of fat, less than 15 g of sugar and less than 0.5 g of salt per 100 g – or, even better, cook fresh foods yourself, so you know what is going into them. Guide them towards nutritious snacks instead of junk food and sweets, and make sure they are getting all the nutrients they need on a regular basis. The basic rules are outlined in the next section.

COMPONENTS OF A HEALTHY DIET

The food we eat is made up of three major kinds of nutrients: proteins, carbohydrates and fats. It also provides the body with vitamins and minerals; these are known as micro-nutrients, because they are required in much smaller quantities. A healthy diet supplies all the nutrients the body needs for it to grow, heal and undertake all the processes necessary to life.

As you'll see from the listings in this book, a single food can combine several different types of nutrients and micro-nutrients. If you eat a varied diet, with the correct number of servings from each food group (see the Food Pyramid on page 44), then you shouldn't need to add up exactly how much you are consuming of each micro-nutrient, but read the list on pages 38-41 and check that you regularly eat foods that supply the main vitamins and minerals.

Protein

Proteins are the building blocks of the human body. The cells of our bones, muscles, skin, nails, hair and every other tissue are made up of proteins. Many vital fluids, such as blood, enzymes and hormones, also contain proteins. There is an enormous variety of different kinds of protein, each made up of a special combination of components called amino acids. The protein in our food is broken down into its component amino acids by the digestive system, and new proteins are synthesized by the body. The best sources of protein in the diet are meat, fish, eggs, milk and other dairy products, tofu, corn, lentils and other pulses. Protein obtained from animal sources contains a greater variety of amino acids than protein from plants. Vegetarians and vegans need to make sure they eat a good mix of legumes, nuts and seeds to get all the amino acids they need, and they should take vitamin B12 supplements if they don't eat dairy.

The Food Standards Agency recommends that protein should represent 15 per cent of the body's daily energy intake, but some experts prefer the guideline that you should eat 0.75 g of protein for each kilogram of body weight. This means that a person who weighs 70 kg should eat 52.5 g of protein. Check the protein column in the listings of this book to find out how much there is in common foods. Athletes might need more than this – maybe 1.2 to 1.4 g per kilo of body weight to build enough muscle. One gram of protein provides about 4 Calories.

In industrialised countries, protein often makes up nearly 40 per cent of the caloric intake. There is little evidence to suggest that too much protein is a health risk, although if it is mainly animal protein, you should watch your cholesterol level (see page 35). However, too little protein is harmful, particularly to the young who are still growing. If you develop white spots on your nails, or brittle, lustreless hair, it could be that you are not eating enough protein.

Carbohydrates

Carbohydrates are the body's main source of energy. They are found mostly in plant-based foods – fruits, vegetables, grains and pulses. Carbohydrates vary in complexity from simple sugars, including glucose, to more complex molecules such as starch and cellulose. Simple carbohydrates, such as the kind of sugar we stir into tea (sucrose) or the sugar found in fruit (fructose), go straight into the bloodstream and give the body a 'lift', but the energy they supply is used up quickly and can cause a feeling of depletion as the blood sugar level drops around 20 minutes later. Many complex carbohydrates are broken down more slowly by the digestive system, giving a steadier blood sugar level and no sense of depletion. The glycaemic index, used on the GI and GL diets, gives carb-containing foods a rating according to their effect on blood sugar, and can be useful for helping to curb hunger and prevent cravings.

Most nutritionists recommend that over 50 per cent of the total daily caloric intake should come from complex carbohydrates. Alternatively, more recent guidelines say you should eat 4–5 g of carbs per kilo of body weight, so a 60 kg person should eat 240–300 g of carb a day. Check the carbs column in the listings to see how many grams of carb are found in common foods. Each gram of carb provides about 4 Calories.

Try to opt for unrefined carbohydrates, such as whole grains, pulses, fruits and vegetables. These are a good source of micronutrients: grains provide B vitamins, while fruit is a good source of vitamin C. Refined carbs, such as white bread, cakes and biscuits, sweets and snacks, have had much of the fibre and nutrient content processed out of them, so energy from these sources is often defined as 'empty Calories'. Also, foods that are high in refined carbohydrates tend to be high in fats as well, and are loaded with Calories.

Some forms of complex carbohydrates are known as dietary fibre. This is not broken down in the digestive tract. It adds bulk to food and contributes to the 'full' feeling after a meal. Although it does not provide any nutrients, it is an essential part of the diet and has a number of beneficial effects, especially assisting the regular and comfortable evacuation of the bowels. Certain kinds of dietary fibre, such as oat bran, are believed to lower levels of cholesterol in the blood.

IN A NUTSHELL...

· Eat fruits and veg of as many different colours as you can each day, to increase the range of vitamins you get.

· Opt for lean protein sources, and keep saturated fats to a minimum.

· Fill up with fibre and drink plenty of water to bulk it up to help the digestive system work efficiently.

The average UK diet provides only about 12 g of dietary fibre a day. Nutritionists recommend that this figure should be nearer 30 g. Check your fibre intake using the fibre column in the listings. Don't increase your intake too rapidly, or it may cause flatulence and diarrhoea; note that very high consumption of fibre may impede the absorption of certain vital minerals.

Fats

Fats in food are the perennial enemy of the dieter. Fat has a very high energy value: 1 g of fat provides 9 Calories, more than twice the calorific value of 1 g of carbohydrate or protein. The fat obtained from food is only broken down and used as energy when other sources of energy – carbohydrate and protein – have been exhausted. If all the fat in the diet is not converted into energy, it is simply laid down in the body's fat stores. A high intake of fats will, therefore, cause weight gain.

There are two categories of fats – saturated and unsaturated. Most saturated fats are of animal origin, although a few, such as coconut oil and palm oil, come from plants. Dripping, lard, butter, cream and cheese all contain saturated fats. Some meats have a high fat content, although this can be reduced by trimming away any visible areas of fat before or after cooking. The liver uses saturated fats to manufacture cholesterol, and high cholesterol can lead to heart disease or strokes when arteries become blocked with cholesterol deposits. To get your cholesterol level tested and find out how your fat intake might affect it, consult your doctor.

Unsaturated fats, found in many vegetable, nut and fish oils, do not raise cholesterol levels and some are thought to actively reduce the risk of heart disease. Olive oil, nuts and seeds, and oily fish, such as mackerel and herring, are especially recommended for the healthy Omega-3 and Omega-6 fatty acids they contain.

Fat represents about 40 per cent of the total energy intake of the average UK diet. This figure is much higher than it needs to be for the body's requirements. We do require some fat as an energy store and for the formation of cell membranes and the protective sheath that surrounds nerves, as well as the synthesis of certain hormones and enzymes. Most fats can be synthesized from excess carbohydrate and protein, but certain essential fatty acids must be obtained from the diet. In order to ensure that these substances appear in the diet, fat should represent at least 2 per cent of the body's energy intake.

However, a diet this low in fat would be unpalatable and difficult to prepare, so nutritionists recommend that fat provides around 20 per cent of the daily intake, with 10 per cent or less from saturated sources. This means that if a person consumes 2,400 Calories a day, 480 of them should be provided by fat in their food. Since 1 g of fat provides 9 Calories, that person should eat about 53 g of fat a day – with a maximum of 26 g of saturated fat.

Fats in common foods

You might be surprised how easy it can be to exceed your recommended daily fat intake. If you have bacon and egg for breakfast along with a slice of buttered toast, you will already have exceeded the recommended fat intake for those on 1,500 Calories per day, and almost all of it is from saturated fat. A hamburger and chips meal plus a Mars bar almost reaches the daily recommended fat intake for someone on 2,500 Calories a day and once again, it's heavily weighted towards unhealthy saturated fat. Using low-fat dairy products and choosing cooking methods other than frying (see pages 42-4) will significantly reduce your intake of saturated fats.

Learn how to read food labels. Note that some low-fat foods have extra sugar added to make them more

Food	Calories	Fat (g)
Whole milk (250 ml)	165	9.75
Semi-skimmed milk (250 ml)	115	4.25
Skimmed milk (250 ml)	80	0.5
Cheddar cheese (30 g)	115	9
Feta cheese (30 g)	75	6
Cottage cheese (30 g)	30	1.29
Low-fat cottage cheese (30 g)	24	0.45
Plain whole milk yoghurt (30 g)	24	0.9
Plain low-fat yoghurt (30 g)	17	0.3
Butter (10 g)	74	8.2
Margarine, soft (10 g)	73	8.1
1 medium fried egg	179	13.9
1 medium boiled egg	147	10.8
Chips, deep-fried (100 g)	280	15.5
Chips, oven-baked (100 g)	162	4.2
Mars bar	449	17.4
Doughnut	262	11.9
Hamburger (each)	253	7.7
Grilled bacon, 2 rashers	295	22

palatable, so they may contain more Calories than non-low-fat alternatives. The term 'fat-free' can be applied to foods containing less than 0.15 g of fat per 100 g – but the term '90 per cent fat-free' means that the product actually has 10 per cent fat. 'Virtually fat-free' means the food contains less than 0.3 g fat per 100 g. 'Low-fat' means it contains less than 3 g per 100 g. 'Reduced fat' means the food contains 25 per cent less fat than the standard equivalent product. Steer clear of trans or hydrogenated fats, found in processed foods, which are associated with high cholesterol levels and increased risk of heart disease.

Vitamins and minerals

Vitamins and minerals are needed by the body in small amounts to enable it to grow, develop and function. A diet that has plenty of fresh, unrefined foods should provide an adequate supply. Many of the processes used to preserve food, such as freezing and canning, can result in loss of nutrients, though, and fruits and vegetables lose some of their goodness every extra day they sit in a fruit bowl or vegetable basket.

Here are the main vitamins and minerals and the foods that are good sources of each. Before you embark on a diet, make sure it will include items from each of these or you may risk suffering from a deficiency.

Vitamin A

- Eggs, butter, fish oils, dark green and yellow fruits and vegetables, liver.
- *Essential for:* strong bones, good eyesight, healthy skin, healing.

Vitamin B1 (Thiamine)
- Plant and animal foods, especially wholegrain products, brown rice, seafood and beans.
- *Essential for:* growth, nerve function, convertion of blood sugar into energy.

Vitamin B2 (Riboflavin)
- Milk and dairy produce, green leafy vegetables, liver, kidneys, yeast.
- *Essential for:* cell growth and reproduction, production of energy.

Vitamin B3 (Niacin)
- Meats, fish and poultry, wholegrains, peanuts and avocados.
- *Essential for:* digestion, energy, the nervous system.

Vitamin B5 (Pantothenic acid)
- Organ meats, fish, eggs, chicken, nuts and wholegrain cereals.
- *Essential for:* strengthening immunity to disease and fighting infections, healing wounds.

Vitamin B6 (Pyridoxine)
- Meat, eggs, wholegrains, yeast, cabbage, melon, molasses.
- *Essential for:* a healthy immune system, production of antibodies, white blood cells and new cells.

Vitamin B12 (Cyanocolbalamin)
- Fish, dairy produce, beef, pork, lamb, organ meats, eggs and milk.

- *Essential for*: energy and concentration, production of red blood cells, growth in children.

Vitamin C
- Fresh fruit and vegetables, potatoes, leafy herbs and berries.
- *Essential for:* healthy skin, bones, muscles, healing, eyesight and protection from viruses.

Vitamin D
- Milk and dairy produce, eggs, fatty fish.
- *Essential for:* healthy teeth and bones, vital for growth.

Vitamin E
- Nuts, seeds, eggs, milk, wholegrains, leafy vegetables, avocados and soya.
- *Essential for:* absorption of iron and essential fatty acids, slowing the ageing process by protecting cells, increasing fertility.

Vitamin K
- Green vegetables, milk products, apricots, wholegrains, cod liver oil.
- *Essential for*: blood clotting.

Calcium
- Dairy produce, leafy green vegetables, salmon, nuts, root vegetables, tofu.
- *Essential for*: strong bones and teeth, hormones and muscles, blood clotting and the regulation of blood pressure.

LOOK FOR THE RDA

If you are unable to get fresh food, look out for
foods that have extra vitamins or minerals added,
such as fortified cereals and breads. Packaged foods
often state the quantity of nutrients and micro-
nutrients they contain, and the percentage they
supply of the EC recommended daily allowance of
each (the RDA).

Iron

- Liver, kidney, cocoa powder, dark chocolate, shellfish,
  pulses, dark green vegetables, egg yolks, red meat,
  beans, molasses.
- *Essential for*: supply of oxygen to the cells and healthy
  immune system.

Magnesium

- Brown rice, soya beans, nuts, wholegrains, bitter
  chocolate, legumes.
- *Essential for*: transmission of nerve impulses,
  development of bones, growth and repair of cells,
  functioning of enzymes and metabolism in general.

Potassium

- Avocados, leafy green vegetables, bananas, fruit and
  vegetable juices, potatoes and nuts.
- *Essential for:* maintaining water balance, nerve and
  muscle function.

Drinks

Water is essential for our bodies to absorb the vital nutrients from our food. It also bulks up the food, stretching the stomach wall and sending that vital message to our brains that we are full, and don't need to eat any more. Water helps the digestive system to flush away waste products; if you suffer from constipation, drinking more water could make a difference. Research suggests we need 1 ml of fluid per Calorie we consume, so if you are on a 2000-Calorie-a-day diet, you should drink 2 litres of water. Some of this will come from fruits, vegetables, soups, softs drinks, tea and coffee, but you will need to top it up with plain water as well.

Remember that alcohol dehydrates you – as well as bumping up your Calorie total without providing any

---

SALT

Excess salt in the diet raises blood pressure and increases the risk of heart disease and stroke. In the UK we consume around 9 g a day, most from processed foods rather than extra salt sprinkled at the table. Experts recommend reducing salt intake to 1.5 g a day and choosing sea salt for its mineral content.

nutritional value. If you drink two small (125 ml) glasses of wine a day, you're consuming 164–190 empty Calories. Two bottles of lager stacks up to 290 Calories, and a double measure of gin with tonic comes to 184 Calories. Drink extra water during and after drinking alcohol to avoid the effects of dehydration (which are one of the causes of hangovers).

Cooking methods

The way you cook food will affect its Calorie content and its nutritional value.

- Any fats added during cooking, such as oil for frying or a knob of butter on top, will add to the Calories in the prepared dish. Young boiled carrots contain 22 Calories per 100 g. A small knob of 5 g butter on top would add another 37 Calories.

- If you boil vegetables, vitamins and minerals leach out into the cooking water; steaming, stir-frying or cooking briefly in a microwave retains more of them.

- Sugar added during cooking will increase Calorie and carbohydrate content. 100 g of apples stewed without sugar have just 35 Calories, while 100 g stewed with sugar have more than double the amount, at 74 Calories.

- Soups, stews and casseroles preserve more of the nutritional value of foods, as vitamins and minerals will be retained in the broth.

- Grilling meat on a grill tray that allows fat to drip through will reduce the fat content. A fried rump steak has 190 Calories per 100 g, while grilled rump steak has only 168 Calories per 100 g.
- In general, the shorter the cooking time, the more nutrients will be retained, and the fewer fats or sugars added, the lower the Calorie count.

The Food Pyramid

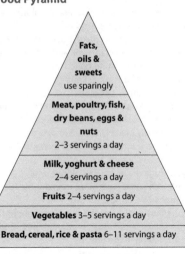

Fats, oils & sweets use sparingly

Meat, poultry, fish, dry beans, eggs & nuts 2–3 servings a day

Milk, yoghurt & cheese 2–4 servings a day

Fruits 2–4 servings a day

Vegetables 3–5 servings a day

Bread, cereal, rice & pasta 6–11 servings a day

When following the Food Pyramid as a guide to healthy eating, it is not necessary to weigh and measure every last crumb but you should bear in mind the following guidelines to portion sizes.

A single serving is not a bowl heaped full of pasta, or a steak the size of a dinnerplate. Portion sizes in restaurants and fast-food outlets have increased almost eight-fold over the past 20 years, as our appetites – and waistlines – have increased. However, the portion sizes indicated on packaged foods may be very small in comparison, and it can be easy to eat more while kidding yourself that you're only consuming the 'Calories per portion' listed on the pack. No wonder consumers are confused!

Remember that every component of a meal or snack must be included in your calculations. For example, a tuna fish sandwich made with two slices of buttered bread would consist of 2 servings of bread, 1 of fish and one of fat.

A serving of fruit is:
· a medium apple or orange (200 g; about the size of a tennis ball)
· a medium banana (150 g peeled; it should fit on the average side plate)

- a half cup (100 g) of chopped fruit or berries
- quarter of a cup of fruit juice.
  A serving of bread, cereal, rice or pasta is:
- 1 slice of bread or ½ bagel or roll
- 30 g of cereal (this will go about halfway up a standard-sized cereal bowl)
- 50 g of cooked rice or pasta (a pile about the size of a child's clenched fist); see the note below.
  A serving of vegetables is:
- a cup of raw, leafy greens (a pile about the size of a woman's clenched fist)
- quarter of a cup of vegetable juice
- a large piece of broccoli (about the size of a lightbulb)

PASTA, RICE AND PULSES

Note that pasta, rice and pulses swell to up to approx. three times their weight when cooked. *The Calorie Counter* gives values for cooked items, while food packaging may often give values for their dry weight. Therefore, 100 g of boiled white rice has 138 Calories, but 100 g of dry uncooked rice has 343 Calories. 100 g of standard cooked pasta has 89 Calories, while 100 g of dried, uncooked pasta has 362 Calories.

- a half cup of chopped vegetables (about as much as you can fit in the palm of your hand)
- 1 baked potato (about the size of a computer mouse).

A serving of milk, yoghurt or cheese is:
- 1 cup (236 ml) of milk or yoghurt
- 28 g of cheese (the volume of four stacked dice, or about the size of your thumb)
- a slice of cheese (the size of a floppy computer disk)
- a half cup (57 g) of cottage cheese.

A serving of meat, poultry, fish, dry beans, eggs, nuts is:
- 85 g lean cooked meat, poultry or fish (the size of a deck of playing cards – or this book)
- 1 medium pork chop
- 1 small hamburger
- 1 fish fillet
- half of a whole chicken breast or a medium chicken leg
- 1 medium egg
- half a cup cooked beans
- 2 tablespoons of peanut butter (roughly the size of a golf ball)
- a handful of nuts or seeds

HOW TO USE THE CALORIE COUNTER

The foods in this book are grouped into categories – Bakery, Biscuits, Burgers, etc – and listed in bold type in alphabetical order in the left-hand column of each page together with the name of the manufacturer of branded foods. The energy value in Calories, the protein, carbohydrate, fat and dietary fibre contents per 100 grams or 100 millilitres are given in the third, fourth, fifth, sixth and seventh columns respectively. This figure has been chosen for convenience but please note that it does not necessarily correspond to the portion sizes described on pages 45-7. To find the values for a 28 g portion of cheese, you would have to divide the figures given by 100 and multiply by 28. Where we have been unable to obtain the information per 100 g/100 ml, it has been specified.

Values for unbranded foods have been obtained from *The Composition of Foods* (5th edition, 1991 and 6th summary edition, 2002) and *Vegetables, Herbs and Spices* (supplement, 1991), and have been reproduced by permission of Controller of Her Majesty's Stationery Office. Where we had gaps, Asda kindly supplied information. We also wish to thank the staff in various branches of Asda, Farm Foods, Holland & Barrett, Sainsburys and Tesco for their assistance.

The recipes in the Family Favourites have been reproduced from *The Composition of Foods 6th Summary Edition* by permission of Controller of Her Majesty's Stationery Office. The aim of including the recipes in this was to allow readers to see where the information was derived from. They were not intended for use as recipes.

The publishers are grateful to all the manufacturers who gave information on their products. The list of foods included is as up-to-date as it was possible to make it, but it should be remembered that new food

CONVERSION CHART

METRIC TO IMPERIAL

100 grams (g) = 3.53 ounces (oz)

1 kilogram (kg) = 2.2 pounds (lb)

100 millilitres (ml) = 3.38 fluid ounces (fl oz)

1 litre (l) = 1.76 pints

1 centimetre (cm) = 0.394 inches (in)

1 metre (m) = 3.28 feet (ft)

Imperial to metric

1 ounce (oz) = 28.35 grams (g)

1 pound (lb) = 453.60 grams (g)

1 stone (st) = 6.35 kilograms (kg)

1 fluid ounce (fl oz) = 29.57 millilitres (ml)

1 pint = 0.568 litres (l)

1 inch (in) = 2.54 centimetres (cm)

1 foot (ft) = 0.305 metres (m)

products are frequently put on the market and existing ones withdrawn, so it has not been possible to include everything. If you cannot find a particular food here, you can still, however, obtain guideline figures by finding an equivalent product from one of the other manufacturers listed in the book.

KEY TO READING TABLES	
g	gram
Cal	Calorie (the same as kcal)
kcal	kilocalorie
ml	millilitre
N	the nutrient is present in significant quantities but there is no accurate information on the amount
n/a	not available
Tr	trace (less than 0.1 g present)
as sold	usually refers to mixes, granules, etc, which need to have milk or water added
recipe	indicates that the recipe used to obtain the nutritional information per 100 g can be found at the back of the book

BAKERY

All amounts per 100g/100ml unless otherwise stated	Cal kcal	Pro g	Carb g	Fat g	Fibre g

NON-BRANDED BREAD AND ROLLS

Bread

	Cal kcal	Pro g	Carb g	Fat g	Fibre g
brown	**207**	7.9	42.1	2	5
brown, toasted	**272**	10.4	56.5	2.1	7.1
ciabatta	**271**	10.2	52	3.9	3.3
currant	**289**	7.5	50.7	7.6	n/a
currant, toasted	**323**	8.4	56.8	8.5	4.2
French stick	**263**	9	56.1	1.9	3.3
garlic bread, pre-packed, frozen	**365**	7.8	45	18.3	N
granary	**237**	9.6	47.4	2.3	5.3
malt, fruited	**295**	7.8	64.9	2.3	3.5
pitta, white	**255**	9.1	55.1	1.3	2.3
rye	**219**	8.3	45.8	1.7	n/a
wheatgerm	**220**	11.1	39.5	3.1	5.7
wheatgerm, toasted	**271**	12.1	53.2	2.6	6.5
white (sliced)	**219**	7.9	46.1	1.6	2.5
white, fried in oil/lard	**498**	8.1	46.8	32.2	2.5
white, toasted	**267**	9.7	56.2	2	3
wholemeal	**217**	9.4	42	2.5	7
wholemeal, toasted	**255**	11.2	49.2	2.9	8.2

Rolls

	Cal kcal	Pro g	Carb g	Fat g	Fibre g
brown, crusty	**255**	10.3	50.4	2.8	n/a
brown, soft	**236**	9.9	44.8	3.2	4.3
hamburger buns	**264**	9.1	48.8	5	n/a
white, crusty	**262**	9.2	54.9	2.2	2.9
white, soft	**254**	9.3	51.5	2.6	2.6
wholemeal	**244**	10.4	46.1	3.3	5.5

All amounts per 100g/100ml unless otherwise stated	Cal kcal	Pro g	Carb g	Fat g	Fibre g
BRANDED BREAD AND ROLLS					
Bagels MR BAGEL'S					
bran & seed	**220**	10.6	43.2	2	9.7
plain	**258**	11.2	52.3	1.7	2.9
plain, mini	**258**	11.2	52.3	1.7	2.9
Bread					
All in One WARBURTON	**216**	8.5	45.9	1.8	7.7
Amazing Grain NIMBLE	**239**	10.7	44.7	1.9	4.7
Best of Both HOVIS	**218**	9.6	39.6	2.3	4.6
brown, crusty HOVIS	**228**	8.7	44.4	1.8	4
Brown Rice ENER-G BREAD	**334**	2.7	45.9	15.5	1.8
Classic White HOVIS	**233**	8.8	44	1.3	2.7
Country Gold Moreishly Malted KINGSMILL	**232**	8.7	43.1	2.7	3.5
Country Grain Multi Seeded HOVIS	**226**	9.8	41.3	2.4	3.6
Country Sandwich HOVIS	**227**	9.7	43.4	1.6	2.7
Danish brown WEIGHT WATCHERS	**213**	11.1	38.9	1.9	7.2
Danish malted WEIGHT WATCHERS	**241**	12.3	44.5	1.7	4.3
Danish white WARBURTON	**243**	10.7	46.9	1.6	2.3
Danish white WEIGHT WATCHERS	**237**	10.5	45.7	1.4	2.3
Danish wholemeal WARBURTON	**229**	13.1	38.6	2.5	7.2
Farmhouse White HOVIS	**224**	8.8	43.9	1.4	2.7
Farmhouse Wholemeal HOVIS	**214**	11	37.8	2.1	6.2
Gold Cosy White KINGSMILL	**239**	8.2	44.5	3.1	2.7
Healthy Inside Wholemeal WARBURTON	**230**	10.8	41.2	2.4	7.5

All amounts per 100g/100ml unless otherwise stated	Cal kcal	Pro g	Carb g	Fat g	Fibre g
Granary HOVIS	**235**	9.4	45.6	1.7	3.8
HiBran ALLINSON	**213**	13.2	33.7	2.8	7.9
Hi-Bran BURGEN	**214**	13.2	33.5	3	7.9
Malted Batch WARBURTON	**262**	10.9	48.8	2.6	5.1
Mighty White Softgrain MIGHTY WHITE	**219**	7.7	43.7	1.5	4.4
Oat Batch	**240**	9.3	42.7	3.5	5.4
Oat Danish WEIGHT WATCHERS	**227**	10.7	38.6	3.3	7.7
Oatmeal CROFTERS KITCHEN	**234**	8.1	41.6	3.9	3.7
Original Wheatgerm HOVIS	**199**	11.5	32.7	2.5	3.7
Premium Brown WARBURTON	**244**	10.3	42.7	3.6	5.1
Rye with sunflower seeds, organic SUNNYVALE	**198**	5.1	30.3	6.3	n/a
Scottish Plain Batch SUNBLEST	**233**	10.1	42.3	2.6	2.8
Seeded Batch WARBURTON	**275**	11.2	38.8	8.4	3.2
Square Cut White HOVIS	**226**	8.9	43.7	1.8	2.8
Square Cut White KINGSMILL	**230**	8.1	44.6	2.1	2.8
Soya & Linseed Bread BURGEN	**274**	15.9	29.8	10.1	6.8
Stoneground Wholemeal WARBURTON	**217**	9.8	39.3	2.3	7.2
Sunflower Maltigrain ALLINSON	**240**	9.8	39.6	4.7	3.9
Sunny HOVIS	**271**	10.1	43.6	6.2	2.4
Tasty Wholemeal KINGSMILL	**220**	10.7	37	3.2	6.8
Toastie Wholemeal KINGSMILL	**224**	10.4	35.8	4.4	7.0
Wheatgerm VITBE	**232**	10.4	39.6	3.6	4.2
white KINGSMILL	**232**	8.8	43.8	2.4	2.8
white MOTHERS PRIDE	**225**	9	45	1	2
white NIMBLE	**245**	9.9	46.4	2.2	2.1

All amounts per 100g/100ml unless otherwise stated	Cal kcal	Pro g	Carb g	Fat g	Fibre g
white SUNBLEST	**228**	8	45.7	1.5	2.8
white WEIGHT WATCHERS	**231**	10.6	43.6	1.6	3.6
White Farmhouse WARBURTON	**236**	9.9	43.4	2.5	2.7
White Granary HOVIS	**249**	11	42	4.1	3.7
White Toastie KINGSMILL	**234**	9.3	42.3	3.1	3.1
White Toastie WARBURTON	**240**	10.1	44.3	2.5	2.8
white, crusty HOVIS	**225**	8.3	44.4	1.6	2.6
white, medium slice WARBURTON	**240**	10.1	44.3	2.5	2.8
white, organic HOVIS	**250**	9.9	46.8	2.6	2.7
white, organic WARBURTON	**224**	9.4	41.3	2.3	2.4
Whole & White KINGSMILL	**228**	9	42.3	2.5	4
wholemeal HOVIS	**208**	10.5	36.6	2.2	6
wholemeal NIMBLE	**209**	11.2	37.1	1.7	6.6
Wholemeal Batch with Oatbran Topping ALLINSON	**217**	12.5	34.7	3.1	7.4
Wholemeal Gold KINGSMILL	**222**	10.3	37	3.6	6
wholemeal, medium slice WARBURTON	**234**	10.3	40.1	3.6	7.2
wholemeal, organic HOVIS	**219**	10.4	36.9	3.3	6.1
wholemeal, organic WARBURTON	**222**	10.3	37.8	3.3	7.6
Wonder White KINGSMILL	**223**	8.4	41.5	2.6	5.3
Chapatis					
made with fat	**328**	8.1	48.3	12.8	n/a
made without fat	**202**	7.3	43.7	1	n/a
plain PATAK	**273**	9.4	48.8	7.5	n/a
Milk Roll WARBURTON White	**249**	11	45	2.8	2.4
Wholemeal	**231**	12.5	38.1	3.2	7

All amounts per 100g/100ml unless otherwise stated	Cal kcal	Pro g	Carb g	Fat g	Fibre g
Naan Bread	**285**	7.8	50.2	7.3	2.9
garlic & coriander SHARWOOD	272	8.5	42.9	7.4	2.4
spicy tomato PATAK	296	8.8	45.2	8.9	n/a
parathas SHARWOOD	277	7.6	41.3	9	1.4
peshwari SHARWOOD	257	7.2	45.1	5.3	2.5
plain feast SHARWOOD	272	8.5	42.9	7.4	2.4
tandoori SHARWOOD	272	8.5	42.9	7.4	2.4
Pitta Bread plain	**250**	10	50	1	3
Rolls					
Best of Both HOVIS	238	10.7	37.4	5	4.2
brown MORTONS	249	11.6	48.9	0.8	5.6
brown SUNBLEST	230	9.7	43.5	1.9	4.3
brown WEIGHT WATCHERS	212	12.1	36.8	1.9	6.3
finger rolls SUNBLEST	253	8.7	47.6	3.1	2.3
Gold Premium White KINGSMILL	240	8.6	43.8	3.4	3.1
Granary HOVIS	273	10	47.3	4.6	4
Granary White HOVIS	296	12	42.7	8.5	3.7
Malted White	251	11.7	47.1	1.8	4.2
Sandwich rolls, white, sliced					
WARBURTON	248	9.4	42.9	4.3	3.4
Seeded WARBURTON	314	13.3	41.2	10.6	3.4
Tasty Wholemeal KINGSMILL	236	10.7	39.2	4	7.4
Tasty Wholemeal WARBURTON	231	10.2	39.1	3.8	n/a
traditional hand made MORTONS	274	11.6	55.3	0.7	1.4
well fired MORTONS	272	11.6	54.2	1	1.7
white HOVIS	251	9.1	43.9	4.4	2.4
white KINGSMILL	250	9.3	44	4.1	2.9

All amounts per 100g/100ml unless otherwise stated	Cal kcal	Pro g	Carb g	Fat g	Fibre g
white MORTONS	**272**	11.6	54.2	1	1.7
white SUNBLEST	**239**	8.9	47.3	1.6	2.3
white WEIGHT WATCHERS	**231**	10.6	43.6	1.6	3.6
white batch WARBURTON	**246**	9.6	42.7	4.1	2.7
White Farmhouse WARBURTON	**250**	9.7	43	4.4	4.4
Whole & White KINGSMILL	**251**	9.5	43.7	4.2	3.5
wholemeal, golden HOVIS	**231**	11.6	36.4	4.3	6.1
Taco Shells OLD EL PASO	**506**	7	61	26	n/a
DISCOVERY FOODS	**448**	n/a	51	24.1	n/a
Tortillas					
corn OLD EL PASO	**343**	10	60	7	n/a
flour OLD EL PASO	**323**	9	52	9	n/a
flour, salsa flavour OLD EL PASO	**343**	10	60	7	n/a
garlic & coriander DISCOVERY FOODS	**313**	n/a	53.9	7	n/a
gluten-free, corn DISCOVERY FOODS	**243**	n/a	53.8	2.3	n/a
plain DISCOVERY FOODS	**313**	n/a	53.9	7	n/a

BREAKFAST & TEATIME BREADS/CAKES

Bagels, cinnamon & raisin					
MR BAGEL'S	**243**	10.9	55.6	2.2	3
Brioche	**347**	8	55	10.5	2.2
Chelsea Buns	**368**	7.8	55.8	14.2	n/a
SUNBLEST	**297**	6.1	52.5	7	2.9
Croissants	**373**	8.3	43.3	19.7	3.1
LA BOULANGÈRE	**410**	8	45	22	n/a

All amounts per 100g/100ml unless otherwise stated	Cal kcal	Pro g	Carb g	Fat g	Fibre g
Crumpets KINGSMILL	180	6.1	37.2	0.8	1.7
SUNBLEST	190	6	39.3	1	2.6
WARBURTON	181	5.9	31.7	0.7	3
Currant Buns	280	8	52.6	5.6	2.9
SUNBLEST	303	6.9	54.7	6.3	2
Danish Pastries	342	5.8	51.3	14.1	N
Doughnuts					
jam	336	5.7	48.8	14.5	n/a
ring	403	6.1	47.2	22.4	N
Eccles Cakes	387	4	56.3	17.8	n/a
Fruit Loaf					
Apple & Cinnamon SOREEN	307	6.9	60.5	4.2	n/a
Lincolnshire Plum SOREEN	302	8.1	57.8	4.3	n/a
Orange & Sultana SOREEN	306	6.8	64.7	4	n/a
Summer Fruits SOREEN	310	7	64.1	4.8	n/a
with Orange WARBURTON	270	7.9	51.7	3.7	3
Hot Cross Buns	312	7.4	58.4	7	n/a
white KINGSMILL	286	7	51.1	6	3
SUNBLEST	291	6.3	52.2	6.3	2.2
Malt Loaf					
fruit, original SOREEN	310	7.4	65.6	2	n/a
Muffins KINGSMILL	224	9.8	42.3	1.7	2.2
SUNBLEST	229	10.2	42.2	2.1	3.3
Chocolate Chip, Micro MCCAIN	447	5.6	51.5	24.2	n/a

All amounts per 100g/100ml unless otherwise stated	Cal kcal	Pro g	Carb g	Fat g	Fibre g
Double Chocolate, Micro McCain	451	6.7	50.4	24.7	n/a
Pancakes Kingsmill	264	6.2	49.7	4.5	1.2
Warburton	329	9	53.4	8.8	n/a
Potato Scones Mother's Pride	207	4.7	42	2.2	4.3
Raisin Loaf with Cinnamon					
Warburton	260	7	50.1	4.1	3.2
Scones					
plain, recipe	364	7.2	53.7	14.8	n/a
Sultana	344	8	51	12	2.9
wholemeal	328	8.8	43	14.6	n/a
Scotch Pancakes	270	5.6	43	9.6	1.9
Sunblest	264	6.2	49.7	4.5	1.2
Soda Scones Mother's Pride	158	4.2	25.4	4.3	3.1
Teacakes					
fruited Sunblest	304	6.9	55	6.3	2.1
fruited Warburton	256	8.7	48	3.3	2.7

CAKES & CREAM CAKES

Almond Slice Lyons Cakes	426	7.1	41.3	25.8	1.6
each Mr Kipling	136	2.3	20.1	5.1	0.7
Angel Slice, each Mr Kipling	155	1.1	22.3	6.8	0.2
Bakewell Slice, each Mr Kipling	150	1.5	19.4	7.4	0.4

All amounts per 100g/100ml unless otherwise stated	Cal kcal	Pro g	Carb g	Fat g	Fibre g
Battenburg Cake LYONS CAKES	**431**	6.9	70.3	13.5	1.3
each MR KIPLING	**161**	1.9	28.1	4.6	0.6
mini, each MR KIPLING	**135**	1.3	25.6	3	0.4
mini, orange & lemon, each MR KIPLING	**133**	1.3	25.3	3	0.4
Buttercream Sandwich LYONS CAKES	**381**	4.4	46.5	19.6	0.7
Bramley Apple Danish Bar SARA LEE	**331**	6.6	41.6	15.6	2.2
Caramel Muffin, Ooh CADBURY	**462**	5.8	50.7	26.2	0.6
Carrot & Walnut Mini Classic, each MR KIPLING	**157**	1.9	18.6	8.3	0.4
Carrot Cake, portion MR KIPLING	**300**	2.4	44.9	12.3	0.9
Corner House LYONS CAKES	**420**	4.7	47.5	23.5	1
Cherry & Almond Cake Bar, each MR KIPLING	**256**	2.8	31.6	13.2	0.8
Cherry Bakewells WEIGHT WATCHERS	**363**	3.6	65.2	11.7	3.2
Chocolate & Orange Cake Bar CADBURY	**433**	4.8	54	22	0.6
Chocolate & Pecan Brownies, each MR KIPLING	**268**	3	31.4	14.5	1.6
Cherry Bakewell Muffin, each MR KIPLING	**437**	5.1	58.5	20.3	1.5
Chocolate Bites CADBURY	**471**	4.6	54.1	26.2	2

All amounts per 100g/100ml unless otherwise stated	Cal kcal	Pro g	Carb g	Fat g	Fibre g
Chocolate Brownies					
McVitie's	**486**	5.1	54.1	27.6	2.1
Ooh Cadbury	**466**	4.9	56.8	24.4	0.5
Chocolate Cake Bars Cadbury	**439**	5.7	55.6	21.6	0.9
Chocolate Chip Bar Cake					
McVitie's	**357**	6.4	57.1	12.5	1
Chocolate Chip Cake Bar					
Cadbury	**434**	5.2	60	23.3	0.8
each Mr Kipling	**151**	1.7	17.1	8.4	0.4
Chocolate Cup Cakes Cadbury	**372**	2.9	69	9.3	0.3
Lyons Cakes	**325**	3.1	68.2	4.4	0.8
Chocolate Digestive Slices					
McVitie's	**467**	4.6	58.5	23.8	2.2
Chocolate Fudge Corner House Cake Lyons Cakes	**373**	3.9	45.3	19.5	0.9
Chocolate Layer Cake Lyons Cakes	**475**	4.8	52.4	27.3	1.6
Chocolate Roll, Rich Cadbury	**387**	4.2	55.7	16.4	1.4
Chocolate Sandwich Lyons Cakes	**384**	3.9	47.9	19.6	1.8
Chocolate Slices, each Mr Kipling	**123**	1.6	14.3	6.7	0.8
Chunky Chocolate Cadbury	**443**	4.3	60.6	23.9	1.2
Chunky Crunchie Cadbury	**491**	4.4	60.6	25.7	0.8
Coconut Hot Cake Lyons Cakes	**364**	4.5	39.9	20.7	1.9

All amounts per 100g/100ml unless otherwise stated	Cal kcal	Pro g	Carb g	Fat g	Fibre g
Coconut Sandwich LYONS CAKES	**408**	3.6	52.3	20.5	1.1
Coffee & Walnut Cake, portion MR KIPLING	**322**	2.9	41.1	16.2	0.7
Coffee & Walnut Cakes, each MR KIPLING	**277**	2.9	28.4	16.9	0.6
Coffee Flavour Sandwich LYONS CAKES	**401**	4.3	53.6	18.8	0.8
Country Slices, each MR KIPLING	**122**	1.4	18.1	4.9	0.4
Date & Walnut Loaf Cake LYONS CAKES	**352**	5.9	41	18.3	1.1
Delectables Chocolate CADBURY	**440**	3.5	52.6	23.9	1
Double Chocolate Muffin, Ooh CADBURY	**448**	5.6	51.1	24.6	0.7
Dream Cake Bars CADBURY	**454**	4.4	56.4	23.4	0.5
Eclairs, frozen	**396**	5.6	26.1	30.6	n/a
Fancy Iced Cakes	**355**	3.8	68.8	9.1	N
Farmhouse Slices LYONS CAKES	**380**	4	58.9	14.2	1.3
Flake Cake CADBURY	**458**	5.4	54.9	24.1	1.3
Flapjack	**493**	4.8	62.4	27	n/a
apricot & sultana, each MR KIPLING	**263**	3.5	30.6	13	2.3
butter, each MR KIPLING	**338**	4	44.4	16.1	2.4
chocolate, Ooh CADBURY	**478**	6.3	59.3	24.1	2.7

All amounts per 100g/100ml unless otherwise stated	Cal kcal	Pro g	Carb g	Fat g	Fibre g
fruit HOLLAND & BARRETT	**468**	4.8	50.8	24.1	n/a
fruit, each MR KIPLING	**306**	3.6	42.3	13.6	2.2
fruit & nut, Ooh CADBURY	**470**	6.8	5.6	24.1	3
Hobnob milk chocolate MCVITIE'S	**454**	5.7	59.5	21.4	4.1
low fat WEIGHT WATCHERS	**364**	6.5	71	6	3.9
plain, wholewheat HOLLAND & BARRETT	**490**	5.3	54.9	27.7	n/a
French Fancies, each MR KIPLING	**106**	0.7	19.6	2.7	0.2
French Sandwich Cake LYONS CAKES	**389**	4	56.4	16.4	0.9
Fruit Cake plain, retail	**371**	5.1	57.9	14.8	N
rich, iced	**350**	3.6	65.9	9.8	N
rich, recipe	**343**	3.9	59.9	11.4	n/a
wholemeal	**366**	6	52.4	16.2	n/a
Fudge Bites CADBURY	**401**	3.9	59	16.6	1.1
Galaxy Cake Bar MCVITIE'S	**497**	5.1	55.8	28.2	0
Gateau, double chocolate	**302**	4.7	28	19	2.7
Ginger Mini Classics, each MR KIPLING	**145**	1.3	18.7	7.3	0.3
Ginger Loaf Cake LYONS CAKES	**347**	5.5	64.1	7.6	1.2
Go Ahead Cake Bar, chocolate dream MCVITIE'S	**394**	4.7	63.9	13.3	0.9
Go Ahead Mini Cake Bars, chocolate chip MCVITIE'S	**356**	6.4	56.9	12.4	1

All amounts per 100g/100ml unless otherwise stated	Cal kcal	Pro g	Carb g	Fat g	Fibre g
Golden Syrup Bar Cake					
McVitie's	385	3.6	60.2	14	1.2
Grannies Cake Lyons Cakes	396	5.3	48.7	20	1.4
Greek Pastries (sweet)	322	4.7	40	17	N
Homebake Cake McVitie's					
chocolate	357	5.7	56.5	14	1.4
lemon	385	4.5	55.5	18	1.1
marble	371	5.2	55.4	14	1.2
Irresistibles Cadbury					
Caramel	457	5.4	60.7	21.4	1.3
Caramel & Nuts	444	5.7	54.8	22.4	1.7
Fudge	407	4	60.4	16.6	1.1
Jaffa Cake Bar McVitie's	408	3.4	58.5	17.5	3
Jamaica Ginger Bar Cake McVitie's	393	3.4	61.9	14.6	1.2
Lemon Cup Cakes Cadbury	284	2.2	48.5	9	0.4
Lemon Drizzle Cake, portion Mr Kipling	279	2.7	44.3	10.1	0.6
Lemon French Fancies, each Mr Kipling	106	0.7	19.8	2.7	0.1
Lemon Luxuries, each Mr Kipling	244	1.6	34.5	11.1	0.3
Lemon Mini Classics, each Mr Kipling	149	1.3	19.6	7.3	0.2

All amounts per 100g/100ml unless otherwise stated	Cal kcal	Pro g	Carb g	Fat g	Fibre g
Lemon Slices LYONS CAKES	383	3.9	61.3	13.5	0.7
each MR KIPLING	120	1.2	18.2	4.8	0.2
Madeira Cake	377	5.4	58.4	15.1	N
Manor House Cake, portion					
MR KIPLING	269	3.9	33.6	13.3	1
Milky Way Cake Bar MCVITIE'S	517	5.3	53.7	31.2	0
Millionaire's Shortcakes, each					
MR KIPLING	356	3.1	40.2	19.2	1
Mini Rolls					
cherry CADBURY	363	4.2	58.8	12.4	0.4
chocolate CADBURY	443	4.4	54.7	22.2	1.3
chocolate WEIGHT WATCHERS	346	4.6	63.9	14.7	3
Jaffa Cakes MCVITIE'S	382	3.5	67.2	11	1.3
strawberry CADBURY	422	3.8	60.4	18.3	0.9
Penguin Snack Cake MCVITIE'S	510	4.8	54.6	30.2	1.6
Raspberry Bar Cake LYONS CAKES	417	4.7	60.7	17.3	1.7
Raspberry Cup Cake CADBURY	284	2.2	48.5	9	0.4
Raspberry Fingers LYONS CAKES	434	3.5	55	22.3	1.9
Sponge Cake					
recipe	467	6.3	52.4	27.2	n/a
dairy cream filled	295	3.7	43	12	0.7
fatless	301	10	53	6.9	n/a
jam filled	302	4.2	64.2	4.9	n/a

All amounts per 100g/100ml unless otherwise stated	Cal kcal	Pro g	Carb g	Fat g	Fibre g
Sticky Toffee Cake Bars, each					
Mr Kipling	**169**	1.8	20	9.1	0.3
Strawberry Sundaes, each					
Mr Kipling	**191**	1.5	28.7	7.9	0.6
Swiss Gateau Cadbury	**404**	4.4	55.7	18.2	1
mini	**449**	4	55	23.6	1.3
Swiss Roll					
chocolate, individual	**386**	4.3	58.1	16.8	N
chocolate Lyons Cakes	**366**	5.4	48.1	16.9	1.4
chocolate, jumbo Lyons Cakes	**397**	4.6	52.4	18.7	1.2
raspberry Lyons Cakes	**292**	5.2	60.5	3.2	1.2
raspberry, per portion Mr Kipling	**184**	1.4	32.6	5.3	0.5
strawberry, jumbo Lyons Cakes	**333**	3.5	51.5	12.5	0.7
Toffee Flavour Loaf Cake Lyons Cakes	**403**	4.8	51.4	19.7	0.9
Trifle Sponges Lyons Cakes	**324**	5.2	67.1	3.9	1
Victoria Mini Classics, each					
Mr Kipling	**149**	1.3	19.6	7.3	0.3
Victoria Slices, each Mr Kipling	**120**	1.4	17.6	4.9	0.4
Victoria Sponge Cake, portion					
Mr Kipling	**285**	3	43.9	10.9	0.8
Viennese Whirls, each					
Mr Kipling	**142**	1.1	15.2	8.5	0.4

All amounts per 100g/100ml unless otherwise stated	Cal kcal	Pro g	Carb g	Fat g	Fibre g

PIES & TARTS

Apple & Blackcurrant Lattice

Tart LYONS CAKES	364	3.4	57.5	13.4	1.5

Apple Pies LYONS CAKES

	384	3.2	57.8	15.5	1.2
MCVITIE'S	235	2.8	35.3	9.6	0.9

Bakewell Tart

LYONS CAKES	397	3.8	56.7	17.2	0.9
MCVITIE'S	396	5	48.9	20	0.7

Bakewell, Cherry, each MR KIPLING	199	1.8	28.4	8.7	0.7

Bakewell, Lemon, each MR KIPLING	208	1.9	30.3	8.8	0.5

Blackberry & Custard Pies, each

MR KIPLING	227	2.4	33	9.5	0.9

Bramley Apple Pies, each

MR KIPLING	229	2.3	36.1	8.4	0.9
individual, each MR KIPLING	493	4.3	79.1	17.8	1.8

Bramley Apple & Blackcurrant

Pies, each MR KIPLING	227	2.3	35.7	8.4	1
individual, each MR KIPLING	490	4.4	78.1	17.8	2.2

Custard Tarts	277	6.3	32.4	14.5	N

Dutch Apple Tart MCVITIE'S	237	3.2	34.4	9.9	0.6

Fruit Pie

individual	356	4.3	56.7	14	N
one crust	190	2.1	28.8	8.2	n/a

All amounts per 100g/100ml unless otherwise stated	Cal kcal	Pro g	Carb g	Fat g	Fibre g
pastry top & bottom, recipe	262	3.1	33.9	13.6	n/a
selection, each MR KIPLING	241	3.4	38.1	8.4	1
wholemeal, one crust	185	2.7	26.5	8.3	n/a
Hot Cross Pies, each MR KIPLING	242	2.5	37.4	9.2	1
Jam Tarts, each MR KIPLING	139	1.3	22.4	4.9	0.5
retail	368	3.3	63.4	13	N
Lemon Curd Tarts LYONS CAKES	406	3.7	59.3	17	1
Lemon Meringue Pie	251	2.9	43.5	8.5	N
HEINZ	294	4.2	47.6	9.6	4.6
SARA LEE	269	2.6	45.1	8.7	1
Mince Pies LYONS CAKES	395	3.7	59.9	15.6	1.5
Red Cherry Pies, each MR KIPLING	241	3.4	38.1	8.4	0.9
Orchards Pie MCVITIE'S	272	3.8	38.4	12	1.1
Treacle Lattice Tart LYONS CAKES	364	4.4	59.3	12	1.1
Treacle Tart	379	3.9	62.8	14.2	n/a

BEANS, LENTILS & CEREAL PRODUCTS

All amounts per 100g/100ml unless otherwise stated	Cal kcal	Pro g	Carb g	Fat g	Fibre g
BAKED BEANS & BAKED BEAN PRODUCTS					
Baked Beans					
in tomato sauce	**84**	5.2	15.3	0.6	n/a
in tomato sauce HEINZ	**72**	4.6	12.9	0.2	3.7
in tomato sauce HP	**85**	4.7	15	0.7	3.7
in tomato sauce, no added sugar WEIGHT WATCHERS	**66**	4.7	11.3	0.2	3.7
in tomato sauce, reduced sugar & salt HEINZ	**66**	4.6	11.5	0.2	3.7
Baked Beans & Vegetable Sausages HEINZ	**105**	6	12.2	3.6	2.9
Baked Beans with Cumberland Sausages HEINZ	**90**	6.4	12.4	1.6	2.9
Baked Beans with Chicken Nuggets HEINZ	**104**	6.6	12.4	3.1	3.2
Baked Beans with Pork Sausages HEINZ	**97**	5.6	11	3.4	3
Baked Beans, curried HEINZ	**96**	4.8	16.3	1.3	4
Barbecue Beans HEINZ	**82**	4.9	14.9	0.3	4
Beef Chilli Baked Bean Cuisine HEINZ	**85**	4.6	10.8	2.6	1.7

All amounts per 100g/100ml unless otherwise stated	Cal kcal	Pro g	Carb g	Fat g	Fibre g
Beef Lasagne Baked Bean Cuisine HEINZ	**90**	5.1	11.5	2.6	1.2
Bolognese Beanfeast, as served BATCHELORS	**62**	5.2	8.1	1	2.1
Cheesy Pasta Bake Baked Bean Cuisine HEINZ	**106**	5	14.3	3.2	1.4
Chicken Casserole with Baked Beans HEINZ	**80**	5.3	11.4	1.5	1.3
Chilli Beanfeast, as sold BATCHELORS	**312**	24.3	42.7	4.9	13.6
Curry Beanfeast, as sold BATCHELORS	**328**	21.1	44.1	7.5	12.5
Lamb Hotpot with Baked Bean HEINZ	**97**	4.8	12.5	3.1	1.7
Mean Beanz HEINZ					
Mexican	**70**	4.5	12.3	0.3	3.6
Sweet chilli	**73**	4.5	13	0.3	3.6
Ocean Pie Baked Bean Cuisine HEINZ	**91**	5.9	10.1	3	1.3
Sausage Hotpot Baked Bean Cuisine HEINZ	**99**	5.2	13.3	2.7	2.5
Savoury Mince Beanfeast, as served BATCHELORS	**75**	6.3	9	1.5	2.3

All amounts per 100g/100ml unless otherwise stated	Cal kcal	Pro g	Carb g	Fat g	Fibre g
Shepherd's Pie Baked Bean Cuisine HEINZ	**88**	4.1	11.6	2.8	1.5
Tuna Pasta Bake Baked Bean Cuisine HEINZ	**103**	6.6	12.8	2.8	1.2

BEANS & LENTILS

Aduki Beans					
dried	**272**	19.9	50.1	0.5	11.1
dried, boiled	**123**	9.3	22.5	0.2	n/a
Blackeye Beans					
dried	**311**	23.5	54.1	1.6	n/a
dried, boiled	**116**	8.8	19.9	0.7	n/a
Broad Beans, canned	**82**	8	11	0.7	5
Butter Beans					
canned	**77**	5.9	13	0.5	n/a
canned BATCHELORS	**83**	6	13.9	0.4	4.8
canned, organic BIONA	**101**	7.1	16.8	0.6	5.2
dried, boiled	**103**	7.1	18.4	0.6	5.2
Cannellini Beans, canned	**87**	7	14	0.3	6
Chick Peas					
canned	**115**	7.2	16.1	2.9	n/a
dried	**320**	21.3	49.6	5.4	n/a
dried, boiled	**121**	8.4	18.2	2.1	n/a

All amounts per 100g/100ml unless otherwise stated	Cal kcal	Pro g	Carb g	Fat g	Fibre g
Chilli Beans					
canned	**80**	4.8	14	0.5	3.7
dried	**70**	4.9	12.2	0.5	3.9
Haricot Beans					
canned	**69**	7	9	0.5	8
dried	**286**	21.4	49.7	1.6	17
dried, boiled	**95**	6.6	17.2	0.5	6.1
Lentils					
green/brown, dried	**297**	24.3	48.8	1.9	n/a
green/brown, dried, boiled	**105**	8.8	16.9	0.7	n/a
red, split, dried	**318**	23.8	56.3	1.3	n/a
red, split, dried, boiled	**100**	7.6	17.5	0.4	n/a
Marrowfat Peas					
canned	**84**	6	14	0.4	4.8
Bigga, canned BATCHELORS	**66**	5.6	10.1	0.3	4
Bigga, dried BATCHELORS	**262**	23.1	37.6	2.1	20.2
Farrow's Giant, canned BATCHELORS	**77**	5.9	12.3	0.5	4.9
quick-soak, dried BATCHELORS	**290**	25.3	41.9	2.4	14
small processed BATCHELORS	**71**	5.4	11.1	0.6	5.1
Mung Beans					
dried	**279**	23.9	46.3	1.1	n/a
dried, boiled	**91**	7.6	15.3	0.4	n/a
Pinto Beans					
canned	**85**	7	13	0.5	8

All amounts per 100g/100ml unless otherwise stated	Cal kcal	Pro g	Carb g	Fat g	Fibre g
dried	**327**	21.1	57.1	1.6	N
dried, boiled	**137**	8.9	23.9	0.7	N
refried	**107**	6.2	15.3	1.1	N
Red Kidney Beans					
canned	**100**	6.9	17.8	0.6	n/a
canned BATCHELORS	**91**	8.1	13.5	0.5	6.4
canned, organic BIONA	**101**	8.4	15.9	0.5	6.7
dried, boiled	**103**	8.4	17.4	0.5	n/a
Refried Beans DISCOVERY FOODS	**85**	n/a	15.1	0.5	n/a
OLD EL PASO	**83**	5.8	13.5	1	n/a
spicy DISCOVERY FOODS	**91**	n/a	16.2	0.5	n/a
Soya Beans					
dried	**370**	35.9	15.8	18.6	n/a
dried, boiled	**141**	14	5.1	7.3	n/a
Split Peas					
dried, boiled	**126**	8.3	22.7	0.9	2.7
yellow, dried WHITWORTHS	**310**	22.1	56.6	1	5.9
Tofu (soya bean curd)					
steamed	**73**	8.1	0.7	4.2	N
steamed, fried	**261**	23.5	2	17.7	N

Fresh beans & peas: *see* **FRUIT & VEGETABLES**

CEREAL PRODUCTS

Barley, pearl, as sold WHITWORTHS	**360**	7.9	83.6	1.7	7.3

All amounts per 100g/100ml unless otherwise stated	Cal kcal	Pro g	Carb g	Fat g	Fibre g
Bran wheat	**206**	14.1	26.8	5.5	36.4
wheat HOLLAND & BARRETT	**206**	14.1	26.8	5.5	36.4
Bulgur Wheat, as sold					
HOLLAND & BARRETT	**357**	12	74	1.4	3.1
Couscous, as sold					
HOLLAND & BARRETT	**355**	13.5	72.5	1.9	2
Cracked Wheat: see **Bulgur Wheat**					
Polenta, ready-made ITALFRESCO	**71.9**	1.6	15.7	0.3	n/a
Wheatgerm	**357**	26.7	44.7	9.2	n/a

BISCUITS

All amounts per 100g/100ml unless otherwise stated	Cal kcal	Pro g	Carb g	Fat g	Fibre g
SWEET BISCUITS					
Abbey Crunch Biscuits McVitie's	**477**	6	72.8	17.9	2.5
Abernethy Biscuits Simmers	**484**	6.6	69.1	21.2	n/a
Boasters McVitie's					
chocolate chunk	**522**	5.9	61.9	27.8	1.8
hazelnut & chocolate chunk	**533**	6.9	52.6	32.8	3.2
Bourbon Creams Jacob's	**467**	n/a	70.4	19.1	n/a
Caramel Digestive Shortcakes McVitie's	**472**	4.5	57.4	24.9	1.6
Caramel Log Tunnock's	**472**	4.2	64.3	24	n/a
Caramel Wafers Tunnock's	**454**	4.6	68	20.1	n/a
dark chocolate	**492**	5.2	60.7	25.4	n/a
Chocolate Biscuit Cakes, gluten-free Itona	**494**	10.9	51.7	27.1	n/a
Chocolate Chip & Orange Biscuits, gluten-free Itona	**467**	10.5	57.6	21.6	n/a
Chocolate Chip Cookies					
Cadbury	**495**	6.5	66.1	22.6	n/a
Chocolatey Cadbury	**485**	7.3	64.3	22.2	n/a
Carb Check Heinz	**457**	7.2	43.1	24.9	7.2
Chocolate Digestive: see **Digestive Bisuits**					
Chocolate Mallow Jacob's	**420**	4.5	65.9	15.4	1.5

All amounts per 100g/100ml unless otherwise stated	Cal kcal	Pro g	Carb g	Fat g	Fibre g
Chocolate Oliver Biscuits FORTTS	**359**	6.5	69.5	23.9	3.9
Chocolate Wafer Cream TUNNOCK'S	**513**	6.6	63.2	28	n/a
Club Biscuits JACOB'S					
fruit	**497**	5.7	61.6	25.3	2.1
milk chocolate	**511**	5.8	62.6	26.4	2
mint	**517**	5.6	62.5	27.2	1.7
orange	**519**	5.6	62.2	27.6	1.7
Coconut Snowballs TUNNOCK'S	**388**	3.9	47	21.8	n/a
Custard Creams					
CRAWFORD'S	**514**	6.1	69.7	23.4	1.6
JACOB'S	**498**	5.3	68.3	22.6	1.4
Date Syrup Biscuits,					
high-fibre ITONA	**387**	10.3	48.2	18.5	12
Digestive Biscuits					
plain	**465**	6.3	68.6	20.3	N
chocolate (milk & plain)	**493**	6.8	66.5	24.1	N
Bournville CADBURY	**490**	6.8	61.6	23.9	n/a
milk chocolate CADBURY	**495**	6.8	62.3	24.4	n/a
milk chocolate MCVITIE'S	**487**	6.7	62.5	23.3	2.9
milk chocolate, light MCVITIE'S	**459**	7.2	68.6	17.3	3.2
plain chocolate MCVITIE'S	**486**	6	61.5	24	4
Double Chocolate Chip Cookies WEIGHT WATCHERS	**445**	4.7	69.7	16.4	5
Fig Rolls JACOB'S	**365**	3.7	69.3	8.1	5.1

All amounts per 100g/100ml unless otherwise stated	Cal kcal	Pro g	Carb g	Fat g	Fibre g
Finger Shortcake McVITIE'S	**464**	5.7	65.1	20.1	2.7
Fingers CADBURY					
caramel	**490**	5.8	63.2	23.8	n/a
caramel, giant	**510**	6	69.8	23.2	n/a
crunchy	**510**	6.6	66.2	23.6	n/a
milk chocolate	**520**	6.8	62.9	26.9	n/a
milk chocolate, giant	**530**	7.5	69	28.5	n/a
white chocolate	**535**	6	61.1	29.7	n/a
Florida Orange TUNNOCK'S	**519**	5.1	64	29	n/a
Fruit & Nut Biscuits, gluten-free ITONA	**461**	11.1	57	20.9	n/a
Fruit & Spice Oat Biscuits, wheat free NAIRN	**424**	7.8	74.6	14.1	8.2
Garibaldi	**397**	5.1	70.8	10.4	2.6
Ginger & Lemon Cookies WEIGHT WATCHERS	**451**	4.2	73.9	15.4	2.2
Gingernut Biscuits	**436**	5.6	79.1	13	N
McVITIE'S	**456**	5.8	70.9	16.5	2.2
Gipsy Creams McVITIE'S	**515**	4.8	66	25.7	2.7
Hob Nobs McVITIE'S	**466**	7.1	60.8	21.7	5.5
milk chocolate	**479**	6.8	60.7	23.3	4.5
milk chocolate, light	**435**	8.1	64.6	16.1	6.2
Jaffa Cakes McVITIE'S	**374**	4.8	70.6	8	2.1

All amounts per 100g/100ml unless otherwise stated	Cal kcal	Pro g	Carb g	Fat g	Fibre g
Jam & Cream Sandwich JACOB'S	**492**	5	67.7	22.3	1.5
Lemon Puff JACOB'S	**516**	6.9	61.6	26.9	2
Lemon Zest Cookies, organic DOVE'S FARM	**435**	3.5	57	21.5	1.9
Lincoln Biscuits MCVITIE'S	**514**	6.3	69	23.6	2
Nice Biscuits	**485**	6.5	68	20.8	2.4
Mixed Berry Oat Biscuits, wheat-free NAIRN	**433**	8	75.6	13.9	6.7
Original Biscuit Cakes, gluten-free ITONA	**496**	12.1	52.2	26.3	n/a
Penguin Biscuit MCVITIE'S	**520**	5.2	62.4	27.7	2.4
Plain Biscuits, gluten-free ITONA	**464**	11.5	58.6	20.4	n/a
Rich Tea Biscuits MCVITIE'S	**453**	7.1	71.2	15.5	2.9
milk chocolate CADBURY	**490**	6.6	67.6	21.4	n/a
Shortbread, recipe	**509**	6	63.3	27.5	N
Shortbread Finger PATERSON'S	**512**	5.3	62	27	1.6
Shortbread Farls TUNNOCK'S	**521**	5.5	62.8	27.5	n/a
Shortcake CADBURY	**500**	6.3	65.8	23.5	n/a
Snack CADBURY					
orange, Sandwich	**525**	7.2	62.6	27.2	n/a
Shortcake	**525**	7	64.2	26.8	n/a

All amounts per 100g/100ml unless otherwise stated	Cal kcal	Pro g	Carb g	Fat g	Fibre g
Shortcake, breakpack	**525**	7	64.2	26.8	n/a
Wafer	**555**	4.3	57.3	33.7	n/a
Stem Ginger Oat Biscuits, wheat-free NAIRN	**439**	7.4	72.8	16.4	7.4
Sultana Cookies, Carb Check HEINZ	**408**	6.9	42.2	20	8
Tea Cakes TUNNOCK'S	**413**	5.3	61	18.1	n/a
dark chocolate	**413**	5.3	61	18.1	n/a
Toffee Cookies WEIGHT WATCHERS	**455**	4.6	72.1	16.5	2.3
Viennese Whirls, each MR KIPLING	**142**	1.1	15.2	8.5	0.4
Wafer Biscuits, filled	**537**	4.7	66	30.1	N
YoYo, mint MCVITIE'S	**545**	3.9	63.1	30.8	1.1

See also: **KIDS' FOOD**

SAVOURY BISCUITS & CRISPBREADS

Allinson Wholemeal Light Crispbread RYVITA	**336**	14.2	66	1.7	12.2
Bath Oliver JACOB'S	**432**	9.6	67.5	13.7	2.6
FORTTS	**412**	8.4	65.5	2.7	n/a
Breaks RYVITA	**333**	8	69.5	2.5	12
Bran Cracker JACOB'S	**454**	9.7	62.8	18.2	3.2

All amounts per 100g/100ml unless otherwise stated	Cal kcal	Pro g	Carb g	Fat g	Fibre g
Butter Biscuits SIMMERS	**483**	6	70	20	n/a
Cheddars JACOB'S	**509**	11.6	53.2	27.2	2.7
Cheeselet JACOB'S	**491**	9.5	55.1	25.8	2.3
Choice Grain Cracker JACOB'S	**419**	8.4	63.4	14.6	7.4
Cornish Wafers JACOB'S	**530**	8	54.4	31.2	2.4
Crackerbread RYVITA					
original	**380**	10.3	76.9	3.5	3.5
high fibre	**321**	12.6	61.3	2.8	16
wholemeal	**319**	10.8	71.5	4.2	6.5
Cream Crackers	**414**	9.5	68.3	13.3	n/a
JACOB'S	**421**	9.9	66.8	12.7	4.1
Croutons					
garlic & herb	**479**	8.4	62.4	25	2.5
slightly sea salted	**491**	8.4	62.2	25	2.7
High Fibre Biscuits ITONA	**406**	8.6	59.4	15	10
Hovis Cracker JACOB'S	**447**	10.2	60	18.5	4.4
Hovis Digestive JACOB'S	**306**	6.2	66.8	18.5	5.8
Krackawheat MCVITIE'S	**515**	9.1	62.4	25.4	4.8
Krispen Crispbread Crackers KAVLI					
light	**371**	10.7	71.8	4.6	5
rye	**272**	10.5	53	2	21
wholemeal light	**366**	9.7	71.2	4.7	7.9

All amounts per 100g/100ml unless otherwise stated	Cal kcal	Pro g	Carb g	Fat g	Fibre g
MacVita wholemeal crackers					
SIMMERS	**447**	8.7	61.6	13.3	11.3
Matzo Crackers RAKUSEN	**367**	9.7	83.8	1.5	2.6
Oatcakes					
black pepper PATERSON'S	**430**	10.6	58.4	17.1	8.1
bran PATERSON'S	**416**	10	58.4	15.8	9.5
cheese NAIRN	**471**	13.4	54	25.1	6.2
fine NAIRN	**455**	10.2	62.5	21.9	8.8
organic NAIRN	**423**	8.8	70.2	16	9.3
rough NAIRN	**429**	11.7	63.5	17.7	7.8
rough PATERSON'S	**430**	10.6	58.3	17.2	8.1
Scottish PATERSON'S	**430**	10.6	58.3	17.2	8.1
Rice Cakes					
original RYVITA	**394**	8.1	83.1	3.2	1.2
sesame	**396**	8.2	82.3	3.8	1.3
Ritz Crackers JACOB'S					
original	**509**	6.9	55.6	28.8	2
cheese	**490**	10.4	55.5	25.2	2.2
Rye Crispbread	**308**	9.4	70.6	0.6	N
Ryvita RYVITA					
original	**315**	8.5	67.2	1.4	16.5
dark rye	**308**	8.5	65	1.5	18.5
multigrain	**332**	11	58.6	6	17.3
sesame	**338**	9.5	60.3	6.5	16.5
Tuc Biscuits JACOB'S	**522**	7	60.5	28	2.9

All amounts per 100g/100ml unless otherwise stated	Cal kcal	Pro g	Carb g	Fat g	Fibre g
Tuc Sandwich Biscuits JACOB'S	**531**	8.4	53.8	31.4	2.3
Water Biscuits					
High Bake JACOB'S	**414**	10.5	76.4	7.4	3
Table CARR'S	**406**	10.1	74.2	7.6	4.2
Wholegrain Crispbread KAVLI					
original	**335**	9.8	70.2	1.7	12.6
garlic	**363**	9.5	69.3	5.2	10.3
onion	**368**	10	67.4	6.5	11.3
Wholemeal Crackers	**413**	10.1	72.1	11.3	4.4

BREAKFAST CEREALS

All amounts per 100g/100ml unless otherwise stated	Cal kcal	Pro g	Carb g	Fat g	Fibre g
BREAKFAST CEREALS					
All-Bran KELLOGG'S	275	14	48	3	27
Alpen Wheat Flakes WEETABIX	350	10.2	72	2.4	9
Apricot Bites KELLOGG'S	279	11	48	3	19
Bran Flakes KELLOGG'S	322	10	66	2	15
yoghurty	352	10	69	4	12
Cheerios NESTLÉ	369	8.1	75.2	3.9	6.6
Honey Nut	374	7	78.3	3.7	5.2
Strawberry	380	8.7	74.7	5.1	5.1
Triple Berry	378	8.7	74.4	5.1	5.4
Choco Crispix KELLOGG'S	383	5	84	3	3
Choco Frosties KELLOGG'S	394	5	80	6	3.5
Chocolatey Squares MORNFLAKE	417	8.3	67.1	12.8	68
Cinnamon Grahams NESTLÉ	411	4.7	76.1	9.8	4.2
Coco Pops KELLOGG'S	383	5	84	3	2
Coco Pops Crunchers KELLOGG'S	380	7	80	3.5	3.5
Cookie Crisp NESTLÉ	378	5.9	80.9	3.4	4.3
Corn Flakes KELLOGG'S	372	7	78	0.9	3
banana crunch KELLOGG'S	408	6	84	8	3
organic DOVES FARM	378	10.3	81.7	1	0.3
Corn Pops KELLOGG'S	382	5	87	1.5	1

All amounts per 100g/100ml unless otherwise stated	Cal kcal	Pro g	Carb g	Fat g	Fibre g
Crunchy Bran Alpen WEETABIX	312	11.5	56.3	4.5	20
Crunchy Nut Clusters KELLOGG'S	435	8	67	15	5
milk chocolate curls	458	8	66	18	4
Crunchy Nut Cornflakes KELLOGG'S	392	6	83	4	2.5
Red	419	7	73	11	3
Nutty	418	7	75	10	2.5
Crunchy Oatbran MORNFLAKE	345	14.8	49.7	9.7	15.2
Fitnesse NESTLÉ	373	6.5	84.5	1	2.4
with fruit	370	6.6	83.4	1.1	3.4
Force NESTLÉ	342	10.6	70.6	1.9	9.2
Frosted Wheats KELLOGG'S	346	10	72	2	9
Frosties KELLOGG'S	371	4.5	87	0.6	2
reduced sugar	369	6	85	0.6	2.5
Fruit 'n' Fibre KELLOGG'S	358	8	68	6	9
Golden Grahams NESTLÉ	375	6	81	3	3.4
Golden Nuggets NESTLÉ	379	6.7	86	1	2.4
Grape Nuts KRAFT	345	10.5	72.5	1.9	8.6
Honey Crispix KELLOGG'S	386	5	88	1.5	1
Honey Loops KELLOGG'S	367	8	77	3	6
Hunny B's KELLOGG'S	379	7	81	3	3
Just Right KELLOGG'S	363	7	48	2.5	4.5

All amounts per 100g/100ml unless otherwise stated	Cal kcal	Pro g	Carb g	Fat g	Fibre g
Malted Wheat Squares, organic					
WEETABIX	**360**	10.8	72.9	2.8	9.3
Multi-Grain Start KELLOGG'S	**375**	8	80	2.5	5
Nesquik Breakfast Cereal NESTLÉ	**381**	7.2	78.8	4.1	4.7
Oat Bran Crispies QUAKER	**383**	11	69	6.5	9
Oat Krunchies QUAKER	**361**	10.5	63	7	11
Puffed Wheat QUAKER	**328**	15.3	62.4	1.3	5.6
Raisin Wheats KELLOGG'S	**325**	9	69	2	9
Rice Krispies KELLOGG'S	**381**	6	87	1	1
Muddles	**371**	8	76	3	8
Ricicles KELLOGG'S	**384**	4.5	90	0.7	0.9
Shredded Wheat NESTLÉ	**340**	11.6	67.8	2.5	11.8
Bitesize	**350**	11.8	69.9	2.6	11.9
Fruitful	**354**	8.3	68.7	5.1	8.9
Honey Nut	**378**	11.2	68.8	6.5	9.4
Triple Berry	**344**	10.6	70.6	2.1	11.1
Shreddies NESTLÉ	**350**	9.9	73.4	1.9	9.8
Coco	**365**	7.6	79.3	1.9	6.9
Frosted	**365**	7.4	80.6	1.4	6.4
Special K KELLOGG'S	**373**	16	75	1	2.5
Red Fruits	**369**	14	76	1	3
Yellow Fruits	**373**	14	77	1	2.5
Yoghurty	**383**	14	75	3	2.5

All amounts per 100g/100ml unless otherwise stated	Cal kcal	Pro g	Carb g	Fat g	Fibre g
Strawberry Squares MORNFLAKE	336	5.8	70.8	3.2	3.5
Sugar Puffs QUAKER	379	5.3	85.8	1.6	3.7
Sultana Bran KELLOGG'S	318	8	67	2	1.3
Sustain KELLOGG'S	360	9	74	3.5	6
Weetabix WEETABIX	336	11.8	68	1.9	10.1
Weetos WEETABIX	384	6.2	78.4	5	5.6

HOT CEREALS

Hot Oat Cereal KELLOGG'S					
Coco Pops	39	7	77	6	4
Fruit 'n Fibre	370	8	71	6	6
Hunny B's	385	7	79	4.5	3.5
Oatbran MORNFLAKE	345	14.8	49.7	9.7	15.2
Oatmeal (Medium or Fine)					
MORNFLAKE	359	11	60.4	8.1	8.5
Oats					
jumbo MORNFLAKE	359	11	60.4	8.1	8.5
organic JORDANS	363	12.5	61.5	7.4	8
organic MORNFLAKE	359	11	60.4	8.1	8.5
porridge JORDANS	363	12.5	61.5	7.4	8
porridge WHITWORTHS	401	12.4	72.8	8.7	7
Quaker QUAKER	356	11	60	8	9
Scott's Piper QUAKER	356	11	60	8	9

All amounts per 100g/100ml unless otherwise stated	Cal kcal	Pro g	Carb g	Fat g	Fibre g
Scott's Porage QUAKER	**356**	11	60	8	9
Superfast MORNFLAKE	**359**	11	60.4	8.1	8.5
Oatso Simple QUAKER					
original	**364**	11	60	8.5	9
apple & blackberry	**364**	7.5	70	6	7
banana	**400**	7	66	12	5
golden syrup	**372**	7.5	71	6	6
raspberry	**396**	7	65	12	5.5
Porridge					
made with water	**46**	1.4	8.1	1.1	n/a
made with whole milk	**113**	4.8	†2.6	5.1	n/a
Ready Brek WEETABIX	**356**	11.6	58.8	8.3	8.9
chocolate	**365**	9.5	65.4	7.3	6.9
Ready Brek Seriously Oaty WEETABIX					
apple & raspberry	**355**	9.5	6.3.7	6.9	6.2
golden honey	**354**	9.4	63.4	7	6.3
thick & tasty	**355**	11.8	57.3	8.7	7.9
Scott's So-easy QUAKER	**364**	11	60	8.5	9
Syrup Swirl	**366**	8	70	6	6.5
Vanilla Cereal, Carb Check HEINZ	**362**	56.7	27.6	2.7	0.4

MUESLI & GRANOLA

Alpen WEETABIX	**362**	10.3	67.2	5.8	6.9
no added sugar	**354**	10.5	64.6	6	7.7

All amounts per 100g/100ml unless otherwise stated	Cal kcal	Pro g	Carb g	Fat g	Fibre g
Alpen, Nutty Crunch WEETABIX	**382**	10.4	66.7	8.2	6.5
Banana & Toffee Crisp MORNFLAKE	**443**	5.7	68.8	16.1	5.4
Chocolate Fruit & Nut Crunch MORNFLAKE	**408**	7.7	66.7	12.3	8.3
Clusters NESTLÉ	**376**	9.4	71.7	5.8	7.3
Country Crisp JORDANS					
apricot	**442**	7.1	65.1	17	7
four nut	**480**	8.9	54.2	25.3	5.9
raisin	**410**	6.2	66.7	13.3	5.9
raspberry	**438**	7.3	64.6	16.7	6
strawberry	**440**	7.3	65.3	16.6	6.9
wild about berries	**443**	7.5	68	15.7	5.7
Country Store KELLOGG'S	**353**	9	68	5	8
Crisp & Flakes Maple & Pecan, organic JORDANS	**436**	8.5	66.2	15.3	5
Crispy Crunch MORNFLAKE	**430**	6.3	70.3	13.7	6
Crunchy Raisins & Coconut Cereal, organic JORDANS	**419**	8.1	66.3	13.5	6.4
Flakes & Clusters JORDANS					
honey nut	**400**	10	61.6	12.5	7.7
maple pecan	**390**	9.4	61.7	11.7	7.7
Fruit & Nut Crunch HOLLAND & BARRETT	**368**	9.8	62.9	9.9	6.4

All amounts per 100g/100ml unless otherwise stated	Cal kcal	Pro g	Carb g	Fat g	Fibre g
Hawaiian Crunch MORNFLAKE	**423**	7.8	66.2	14.1	6.5
Luxury Crunchy Cereal JORDANS					
fruits & nuts	**421**	7	66	14.3	5.5
maple & pecan	**448**	9.9	59.9	18.7	6.5
summer fruits	**340**	7.5	53.5	10.7	6.2
Minis WEETABIX					
banana crisp	**371**	9	71.9	5.3	8.3
chocolate crisp	**378**	9.3	72.3	5.7	7.9
fruit & nut crisp	**362**	9.5	70.3	4.8	8.2
honey & nut crisp	**369**	10.1	72.6	4.2	6.7
Muesli					
apricot HOLLAND & BARRETT	**284**	7.7	59	3.5	5.6
crunchy bran HOLLAND & BARRETT	**352**	8.8	62.9	9.9	6.4
gluten-free HOLLAND & BARRETT	**390**	14.1	54.1	13	3.3
luxury fruit WEIGHT WATCHERS	**318**	7.2	67.7	2	8.1
natural JORDANS	**346**	9.6	63	6.2	8.6
organic JORDANS	**353**	8.9	59.5	8.7	9
original HOLLAND & BARRETT	**351**	11.1	61.2	8.4	7.1
Premium Fruit KELLOGG'S	**345**	8	58	9	11
Rich HOLLAND & BARRETT	**358**	10	60.5	9.2	7.6
Special JORDANS	**384**	9.6	58.4	12.5	8.2
Special Fruit JORDANS	**323**	5.7	68.9	2.7	7.1
Super Cranberry, Cherry & Almond DORSET CEREALS	**329**	10	54.8	7.7	7.5
Swiss style	**363**	9.8	72.2	5.9	n/a
Swiss style, organic JORDANS	**359**	9.7	62.9	7.6	7.4

All amounts per 100g/100ml unless otherwise stated	Cal kcal	Pro g	Carb g	Fat g	Fibre g
Swiss style, special JORDANS	**360**	11.6	64.9	6	8.2
with no added sugar	**366**	10.5	67.1	7.8	n/a
Oat Crunch QUAKER	**445**	8	66.5	16	5
Original Crunchy Cereal JORDANS					
raisins & almonds	**410**	8.4	66	12.5	5
tropical fruits	**424**	9	66	13.8	5
Pecan & Maple Crisp MORNFLAKE	**437**	6.6	67.2	15.7	5.7
Raspberry Crisp MORNFLAKE	**428**	6.5	68.2	14.3	6.8
Strawberry Crisp MORNFLAKE	**436**	6.5	68.9	14.9	6.3
Sultana & Apple Crunch MORNFLAKE	**378**	7.6	59.3	12.2	12.5
Traditional Crunch MORNFLAKE	**400**	8	65.4	11.8	9.6
Treasure Crunch MORNFLAKE	**377**	7.7	60.2	11.7	10.7
Triple Chocolate Crisp MORNFLAKE	**435**	7.1	67.7	15.1	4.9

CEREAL BARS

	Cal kcal	Pro g	Carb g	Fat g	Fibre g
Alpen Apple & Blackberry Cereal Bar,					
with yoghurt, each WEETABIX	**117**	1.6	20.8	3.1	1.5
Alpen Banana & Coconut Cereal Bar,					
with chocolate, each WEETABIX	**119**	2.1	20.1	4.1	0.7
Alpen Fruit & Nut Cereal Bar,					
each WEETABIX	**110**	1.8	19.9	2.6	1
with chocolate, each	**122**	1.9	19.8	3.9	1

All amounts per 100g/100ml unless otherwise stated	Cal kcal	Pro g	Carb g	Fat g	Fibre g
Alpen Papaya & Pineapple Cereal Bar, with chocolate, each WEETABIX	**119**	2	20.6	3.2	1.2
Alpen Raspberry Cereal Bar, with yoghurt, each WEETABIX	**121**	1.6	21.3	3.2	0.9
Alpen Strawberry Cereal Bar, with yoghurt, each WEETABIX	**119**	1.7	21	3.1	1.1
Apple & Sultana Break Bar each JORDANS	**148**	1.9	27.8	3.2	1.9
Apricot & Green Tea Cereal Bar SVELTESSE	**389**	5.4	69.2	9.9	6.9
Brunch Bar CADBURY					
cranberry & orange	**440**	6	68	16	n/a
hazelnut	**465**	7	61	22	n/a
raisin	**430**	6	67	16	n/a
Cereal & Milk Bar KELLOGG'S					
Choco Frosties	**417**	7	68	13	1.5
Coco Pops	**420**	7	67	14	1
Frosties	**380**	8	69	15	1.5
Rice Krispies	**413**	7	68	13	0.3
Chewee, each QUAKER					
milk chocolate chip	**95**	1.2	15	3.5	0.8
Chocolate & Banana Cereal Bars, each, Carb Check HEINZ	**142**	6.1	12	5.5	0.9

All amounts per 100g/100ml unless otherwise stated	Cal kcal	Pro g	Carb g	Fat g	Fibre g
Chunkyfruit Bars WEETABIX					
apple, each	**158**	1.8	31.3	2.9	n/a
blackcurrant & apple, each	**158**	1.8	31.3	2.9	n/a
cherry, each	**158**	1.8	31.2	2.9	n/a
strawberry, each	**158**	1.8	31.2	2.9	n/a
Citrus Burst Cereal Bar SKI	**385**	4.2	70.3	9.7	3
Coconut & Raspberry Cereal Bars,					
each, Carb Check HEINZ	**99**	3.2	8.4	5.4	4.5
Crunchy Bar, each JORDANS					
honey & almond	**131**	2.4	17.9	5.5	2.1
organic	**151**	2.7	18.9	7.2	2.6
Crunchy Nut Cereal Bar KELLOGG'S	**446**	6	69	16	1.5
Fruit & Fibre Cereal Bar KELLOGG'S	**380**	5	71	9	5
Fruit & Nut Break, each JORDANS	**170**	3	23.7	7	2
Frusli Bar, each JORDANS					
blueberry burst	**114**	1.6	20.5	2.9	1.4
cranberry & apple	**114**	1.7	20.2	3	1.5
raisin & hazelnut	**123**	2	18.3	4.6	1.4
tangy citrus	**113**	1.3	20.3	3	1.4
wild berries	**112**	1.5	20.5	2.7	1.6
Go Fruity Cereal Bar, each SOREEN	**144**	2.5	29.2	1.9	n/a
Luxury Bar, each JORDANS					
Absolute Nut	**256**	5.7	9.9	21.5	4.7
Cranberry & Almond	**212**	3.8	29.3	8.9	2.6
Vine Fruit & Nut	**225**	4.3	25.3	11.9	2.1

All amounts per 100g/100ml unless otherwise stated	Cal kcal	Pro g	Carb g	Fat g	Fibre g
Nutri-grain Bar KELLOGG'S					
apple	**353**	4	66	9	3.5
blackberry & apple	**356**	4	69	8	3
blueberry	**351**	4	66	9	4
cherry	**348**	4	67	8	4
chocolate	**367**	4.5	66	10	4
orange	**349**	4	65	9	4
strawberry	**355**	4	67	9	3.5
Nutri-grain Bar Elevenses KELLOGG'S					
Ginger	**373**	5	68	9	3
Raisin	**367**	5	67	9	3.5
Nutri-grain Mini Bars KELLOGG'S					
apple	**350**	3.5	71	7	3.5
blueberry	**363**	4	69	9	3.5
raspberry yoghurty	**361**	4.5	68	9	3.5
strawberry	**363**	4	69	9	3.5
strawberry yoghurty	**361**	4.5	68	9	3.5
Red Berry Cereal Bar SVELTESSE	**389**	5.4	69.2	9.9	6.8
SKI	**386**	4.3	70.2	9.8	3.4
Rice Krispies Squares KELLOGG'S	**406**	3	72	12	0.9
chocolate & caramel	**425**	4.5	73	13	2
Special K Cereal Bar KELLOGG'S	**400**	8	74	8	2
Peaches & Apricot	**400**	8	73	9	2.5
Pear & Apple	**400**	8	73	8	2
Special Muesli Bar, each JORDANS	**193**	3.1	30.7	6.5	2.7

All amounts per 100g/100ml unless otherwise stated	Cal kcal	Pro g	Carb g	Fat g	Fibre g
Sultana & Honey Break, each					
JORDANS	**136**	2.1	23.2	3.9	1.4
Tracker Bar MARS					
chocolate chip	**490**	6.9	59	24.1	1.7
forest fruits	**474**	4.6	64.1	22.2	n/a
lemon	**477**	4.6	64.3	22.4	n/a
roasted nut	**504**	8.9	54.7	26.7	1.4
Weetos with Real Milk Chocolate Cereal Bars, each WEETABIX	**88**	1.2	14.2	2.9	0.3
Weetos Honey with Real Milk Chocolate Cereal Bars, each					
WEETABIX	**87**	1.1	14.5	2.7	0.3

BURGERS

All amounts per 100g/100ml unless otherwise stated	Cal kcal	Pro g	Carb g	Fat g	Fibre g
Beefburgers					
fried	**329**	28.5	0.1	23.9	n/a
grilled	**326**	26.5	0.1	24.4	n/a
100%, each Birds Eye	**120**	9.9	0.1	9.1	0
mega, each Birds Eye	**310**	23	7.1	21	0.5
original, each Birds Eye	**115**	8.3	2.9	7.8	0.2
quarter-pounders, each Birds Eye	**254**	14.6	5.1	19.5	0.4
with onion Ross	**284**	14.7	2.8	23.8	0.4
Chicken Burgers Birds Eye	**140**	7.5	10	7.9	0.5
quarter-pounders, each	**285**	16	22	15	0.3
Cajun fillet burger, each	**130**	21	2.3	3.9	0.2
fillet burger, each	**130**	21	2.7	3.9	0.1
Chilli Beef Quarter Pounders,					
each Birds Eye	**235**	13.9	7.4	16.4	0.9
Lamb Burgers, uncooked Ross	**300**	13.2	3.6	25.9	1.2
Veggie Burgers flame-grilled					
Linda McCartney Foods	**174**	17.9	13.8	5.2	3.3
vegetable burgers					
Linda McCartney Foods	**238**	3.1	27.7	12.7	2.3
Vegetable Quarter Pounders,					
each Birds Eye	**240**	5.4	28	12	2.1

See also: **FAST FOOD**

CHIPS, FRIES & SHAPED POTATO PRODUCTS

All amounts per 100g/100ml unless otherwise stated	Cal kcal	Pro g	Carb g	Fat g	Fibre g
Non-branded Chips					
crinkle cut, frozen, for frying	**168**	2.3	24	7	8
crinkle cut, frozen, oven baking	**134**	2	23	3.8	8
French fries, retail	**280**	3.3	34	15.5	n/a
homemade, fried	**189**	3.9	30.1	6.7	n/a
microwave	**221**	3.6	32.1	9.6	n/a
oven	**162**	3.2	29.8	4.2	n/a
retail	**239**	3.2	30.5	12.4	n/a
straight cut, frozen, fried	**273**	4.1	36	13.5	n/a
Chips, Chip Shop ROSS	**75**	2	17.6	0.2	1.3
Chips, Chunky ROSS	**118**	2.4	21.9	3	1.6
Croquettes, Potato, fried in oil	**214**	3.7	21.6	13.1	n/a
Croquette Royales, Cheesey ROSS	**228**	4.2	23.7	13.4	1.6
Hash Browns MCCAIN	**153**	2.9	26.8	5	n/a
Home Fries MCCAIN	**141**	2	23.2	4.4	n/a
chunky	**137**	2.4	25.1	3	n/a
crinkle cut	**143**	2.1	22.4	4.9	n/a
thin & crispy	**157**	3.1	24.6	5.1	n/a
Home Roasts MCCAIN	**153**	2.9	26.8	5	n/a
French Fries MCCAIN	**134**	2.2	24.9	3.7	n/a
Crispy	**241**	4.2	41.1	8.4	n/a
Mash MCCAIN	**108**	3.1	17.9	2.7	n/a

All amounts per 100g/100ml unless otherwise stated	Cal kcal	Pro g	Carb g	Fat g	Fibre g
Micro Chips McCain	**172**	2.9	28.8	6.3	n/a
crinkle cut	**183**	2.5	31.5	6.6	n/a
Oven Chips					
crinkle cut McCain	**163**	2.9	30.2	5.4	n/a
straight cut McCain	**172**	3.4	32.4	4.9	n/a
Ross	**131**	2.4	20.6	5.1	1.6
Weight Watchers	**110**	2.1	23	2.6	3.1
Oven Crunchies, as sold Ross	**158**	2.5	21	7.1	1.7
Potato Fritters, Crispy, as sold					
Birds Eye	**145**	2	16.3	8	1.2
Potato Pancakes Ross	**239**	3.2	18.8	17.4	1.3
with Onion	**228**	2.9	22	15.2	2.2
Potato Skins Birds Eye					
cheese & bacon	**197**	6.6	21.6	9.3	2.1
cheese & tomato	**143**	4.6	18.9	5.4	2.2
chilli con carne	**110**	3.6	19.7	1.9	2.2
Potato Waffles					
frozen, cooked	**200**	3.2	30.3	8.2	n/a
frozen, cooked Birds Eye	**167**	2	20.7	8.5	1.5
frozen, cooked Ross	**225**	2.3	22	12.3	2
Roast Potatoes Weight Watchers	**91**	2.3	20.5	1.9	2.5
Rosti McCain	**246**	3.1	29.7	12.8	n/a
Southern Fries McCain	**297**	5.3	44.9	10.2	n/a

All amounts per 100g/100ml unless otherwise stated	Cal kcal	Pro g	Carb g	Fat g	Fibre g
Wedges, oven baked McCAIN					
Mexican Chilli	**230**	5.2	37.2	8.8	n/a
Nicely Spiced	**238**	3.7	36.1	10.5	n/a
Sea Salt & Cracked Black Pepper	**214**	3.8	36.9	7.4	n/a
Sour Cream & Chive	**193**	3.5	34.3	6.1	n/a

CONDIMENTS & SAUCES

All amounts per 100g/100ml unless otherwise stated	Cal kcal	Pro g	Carb g	Fat g	Fibre g
TABLE SAUCES					
Apple Sauce BAXTERS	**86**	0.3	21	0.1	n/a
Bramley COLMAN'S	**107**	0.2	26.5	Tr	1.3
Barbecue Sauce, bottled					
HELLMANN'S	**125**	0.8	27.7	0.7	Tr
classic HP	**143**	0.8	33.1	0.2	0.7
hot 'n' sizzly HEINZ	**124**	1.1	28.1	0.4	0.3
hot 'n' spicy HP	**131**	0.9	29.8	0.2	Tr
low carbohydrate CARB OPTIONS	**42**	0.5	8.7	0.1	0.5
original HEINZ	**135**	1	31.3	0.4	Tr
smoky bacon HP	**120**	0.7	28.5	0.2	0.8
spicy HP	**156**	0.9	36.7	0.1	Tr
tangy zest HP	**127**	0.4	32.6	Tr	0.7
Beetroot in Redcurrant Jelly					
BAXTERS	**167**	0.6	41	Tr	n/a
Branston Rich & Fruity Sauce					
CROSSE & BLACKWELL	**121**	1.4	28.5	0.2	n/a
Brown Sauce bottled	**98**	1.2	22.2	0.1	n/a
bottled DADDIES	**102**	0.9	24.3	Tr	0.9
Burger Sauce HELLMANN'S	**240**	1.1	12	21	Tr
Chilli Ketchup HEINZ	**102**	1.2	23.2	0.2	0.5
Chilli Sauce HP	**134**	1.2	32.3	Tr	0.9
Cranberry Jelly BAXTERS	**268**	Tr	67	Tr	0

All amounts per 100g/100ml unless otherwise stated	Cal kcal	Pro g	Carb g	Fat g	Fibre g
OCEAN SPRAY	**136**	0.2	36.2	0.1	0.2
Cranberry Sauce BAXTERS	**180**	0.1	45	0	n/a
OCEAN SPRAY	**158**	0.1	40.8	0.1	1.3
with Orange Liqueur OCEAN SPRAY	**205**	0.3	50	0.4	n/a
Curry Ketchup HEINZ	**104**	1.1	23.7	0.1	0.8
Curry Sauce HP	**124**	1.4	24.2	2.4	2.1
Fruity Sauce HP	**141**	1.2	33.7	0.3	0.9
Garlic Sauce LEA & PERRINS	**337**	1.8	17.8	29	n/a
Horseradish Relish COLMAN'S	**112**	1.9	9.8	6.2	2.6
Horseradish Sauce	**153**	2.5	17.9	8.4	n/a
COLMAN'S	**112**	1.9	9.8	6.2	2.6
HP Sauce HP	**119**	1.9	27.1	0.2	1.3
Mint Jelly BAXTERS	**264**	Tr	66	0	n/a
Mint Sauce BAXTERS	**62**	1.7	13.2	0.3	n/a
BURGESS	**68**	1.6	12	0	2
classic COLMAN'S	**116**	1	25.6	0.2	1.6
fresh garden COLMAN'S	**21**	1.8	3.1	0.2	1.9
Mushroom Ketchup BURGESS	**27**	0.5	5.5	0.1	Tr
Raita with Mint & Cucumber PATAK	**117**	3.9	12.9	5.5	0.1
Redcurrant Jelly BAXTERS	**260**	0	65	0	n/a

All amounts per 100g/100ml unless otherwise stated	Cal kcal	Pro g	Carb g	Fat g	Fibre g
Saucy Chip Dip HELLMANN'S	280	1	10	26	0
Soy Sauce (light & dark)	43	3	8.2	Tr	n/a
Tabasco, per serving (1 tsp)	0	0	0	0	0
Tartare Sauce BAXTERS	516	0.9	8.5	53.1	n/a
COLMAN'S	284	1.2	17	23	0.6
Tomato Ketchup	115	1.6	28.6	0.1	n/a
DADDIES	110	0.9	26.5	Tr	0.9
HEINZ ·	102	0.2	4.8	Tr	0.1
Carb Check HEINZ	58	1.4	11.8	0.1	0.9
low carbohydrate CARB OPTIONS	57	1.4	10.8	0.1	1.8
organic MERIDIAN FOODS LTD	114	1.8	28.4	0.1	1.1
Wild Rowan Jelly BAXTERS	268	0	67	0	n/a
Worcestershire & Tomato Sauce					
LEA & PERRINS	102	0.8	23	0.5	0.7
Worcestershire Sauce LEA & PERRINS	92	0.9	22.2	0.1	0.9

MUSTARDS

Dijon Mustard COLMAN'S	101	5.6	2.3	7.8	2
English Mustard BURGESS	175	7.2	20	6.8	0.5
original COLMAN'S	188	7	19	9.3	1.6
French Mustard BURGESS	144	6.8	12.6	6	0.2
Mild Mustard COLMAN'S	95	4.9	8.4	4.6	4
Wholegrain Mustard COLMAN'S	154	8.8	8.9	9.3	3.4

All amounts per 100g/100ml unless otherwise stated	Cal kcal	Pro g	Carb g	Fat g	Fibre g
VINEGARS					
Balsamic Vinegar CARAPELLI	**100**	Tr	21	0	0
Cider Vinegar DUFRAIS	**20**	0.1	1.2	0	0
HOLLAND & BARRETT	**18**	0	0.1	0	0
Garlic Vinegar DUFRAIS	**20**	0.1	0.8	0	0
Raspberry Vinegar DUFRAIS	**20**	0.1	1	0	0
Red Wine Vinegar DUFRAIS	**25**	0.2	0.8	0	0
Sherry Vinegar DUFRAIS	**25**	0.4	1.7	0	0
Tarragon Vinegar DUFRAIS	**20**	0.1	0.8	0	0
White Wine Vinegar DUFRAIS	**20**	0.1	0.8	0	0
STOCK CUBES, GRANULES & PURÉES					
Aromat KNORR	**165**	13.1	20.8	3.6	1
Beef Gravy Granules with Pink Peppercorn Flavour, as sold OXO	**315**	8.1	59.3	5	0.2
Beef Gravy Granules, Winter Berry & Shallot Flavour, as sold OXO	**320**	7.8	61.3	4.9	2.1
Beef Stock Cubes as sold OXO	**259**	14.9	40	4.4	1.6
prepared BOVRIL	**6**	0.3	0.9	0.1	Tr
prepared KNORR	**7**	0.2	0.5	0.5	Tr
Bisto Original Gravy Powder, as sold BISTO	**257**	2.1	61.9	0.1	0.3

All amounts per 100g/100ml unless otherwise stated	Cal kcal	Pro g	Carb g	Fat g	Fibre g
Bouillion KNORR					
beef	**73**	7.5	9.5	0.5	n/a
chicken	**75**	4	8	3	n/a
fish	**69**	7.5	9	0.3	n/a
vegetable	**101**	7.5	17	0.3	n/a
Chicken Granulated Stock KNORR	**232**	13.1	36.5	3.7	0.4
Chicken Gravy Granules,					
as sold BISTO	**395**	3.5	59.7	15.8	0.2
as sold OXO	**322**	9.7	61.9	4	2.2
with a hint of sage & onion flavour OXO	**316**	11.1	54.2	6.1	0.7
Chicken Stock Cubes,					
as sold OXO	**249**	11.7	42.9	3.4	1.6
prepared KNORR	**7**	0.2	0.5	0.4	Tr
Chinese Herb & Spice Cubes OXO	**274**	9.5	42.9	7.2	3.6
Cracked Black Pepper & Roasted Garlic Flavour Gravy Sauce, prepared BISTO	**50**	0.5	6.2	2.5	0.9
Fish Stock Cubes, prepared KNORR	**7**	0.4	0.1	0.5	Tr
Garlic Purée	**423**	2.7	13	40	6
Gravy Browning BURGESS	**72**	3.3	14.7	0	0
Gravy Granules for Meaty Dishes, as sold OXO	**319**	8.7	61	4.4	0.8

All amounts per 100g/100ml unless otherwise stated	Cal kcal	Pro g	Carb g	Fat g	Fibre g
Gravy Granules for Vegetable, Dishes as sold Oxo	**309**	8.4	59.3	4.2	3.1
Gravy Granules with Onion,					
as sold Bisto	**365**	2.9	56.1	14.3	1.8
Oxo	**365**	2.9	56.1	14.3	1.8
Gravy Instant Granules	**462**	4.4	40.6	32.5	n/a
made up with water	**34**	0.3	3	2.4	n/a
Favourite, as sold Bisto	**385**	2.5	57.3	16.2	1.3
Ham Stock Cubes, prepared					
Knorr	**7**	0.3	0.4	0.4	Tr
Indian Herb & Spice Cubes Oxo	**287**	11.9	43.4	7.3	9.7
Italian Herb & Stock Cubes Oxo	**316**	11.2	49.5	8.1	5
Lamb Gravy Granules, garden mint flavour, as sold Oxo	**349**	9.6	60.3	7.7	1
Lamb Stock Cubes					
prepared Knorr	**7**	0.3	0.1	0.5	Tr
as sold Oxo	**291**	12.6	51.2	4	1.7
Marmite Stock Cubes Bestfoods	**247**	25	25.5	5	n/a
Mexican Herb & Spice Cubes Oxo	**292**	8.2	46.2	8.3	2.7
Onion Gravy Granules with a hint of sage & thyme Oxo	**319**	5.7	63.8	4.5	2.5
Pork Stock Cubes, prepared Knorr	**7**	0.3	0.3	0.5	Tr

All amounts per 100g/100ml unless otherwise stated	Cal kcal	Pro g	Carb g	Fat g	Fibre g
Roast Onion & Ale Gravy Flavoured Sauce, prepared BISTO	**45**	0.5	6.8	1.7	0.7
Roast Vegetable Flavour Gravy Granules, as sold BISTO	**317**	2.1	64.2	5.7	1.1
Rosemary & Red Wine Gravy Flavoured Sauce, prepared BISTO	**45**	0.3	6.9	1.8	0.9
Tomato Purée	**76**	5	14.2	0.3	n/a
NAPOLINA	**90**	4.8	18	Tr	n/a
Vegetable Granulated Stock KNORR	**199**	8.5	39.9	0.6	0.9
Vegetable Stock Cubes, prepared KNORR	**10**	0.3	0.3	0.9	Tr
as sold OXO	**258**	9.8	45.3	4.2	1.7
White Sauce Granules, as sold BISTO	**480**	3.3	54.1	27.9	2.5

STUFFINGS

Apple, Mustard & Herb Stuffing Mix PAXO	**166**	4.2	32.8	2	4
Chestnut & Cranberry Stuffing Mix PAXO	**141**	4	26.7	2	2.4
Redcurrant & Rosemary Stuffing Mix, PAXO	**123**	3.5	23	1.9	3

All amounts per 100g/100ml unless otherwise stated	Cal kcal	Pro g	Carb g	Fat g	Fibre g
Crumb Dressing RUSKOLINE	**333**	10.5	69	1.7	4.6
Parsley, Thyme & Lemon Stuffing Mix PAXO	**97**	2.7	19.4	1	1.8
Sage & Onion Stuffing	**269**	6.1	29	15.1	n/a
WHITWORTHS	**398**	5.7	73.6	9	1.9
Sage & Onion Stuffing Mix PAXO	**123**	3.6	23	1.8	1.7
Sausagemeat & Thyme Flavour Stuffing Mix PAXO	**160**	6.3	25.8	3.5	4

DRESSINGS

Blue Cheese Dressing	**457**	2	8.7	46.3	n/a
Blue Cheese Flavoured Low Fat Dressing WEIGHT WATCHERS	**59**	1.5	5.8	3.4	0
Caesar Dressing HELLMANN'S	**494**	2.5	3.5	52.2	0.3
Creamy KRAFT	**335**	3	7.9	32	0.2
Light KRAFT	**102**	2.1	15	3.5	0.1
low carbohydrate CARB OPTIONS	**467**	2.4	1.3	50	0.8
low fat, Waistline CROSSE & BLACKWELL	**128**	1.1	10.5	9.1	n/a
warm HELLMANN'S	**538**	4.5	7.9	54.2	1.4
Caesar Style Low Fat Dressing WEIGHT WATCHERS	**80**	3.3	14.7	0.9	0.2
Chinese Warm Dressing HELLMANN'S	**141**	2	13.6	8.7	1.5

All amounts per 100g/100ml unless otherwise stated	Cal kcal	Pro g	Carb g	Fat g	Fibre g
Creamy Dressing, Waistline					
CROSSE & BLACKWELL	124	0.8	15.1	6.7	n/a
French Dressing					
recipe	462	0.1	4.5	49.4	0
HELLMANN'S	297	0.4	14.9	25.9	0.3
Classic KRAFT	159	0.9	7.3	13.5	0.1
Light KRAFT	39	0.1	8.7	Tr	0.5
low carbohydrate CARB OPTIONS	233	0.2	0.8	25.3	0.8
organic MERIDIAN FOODS LTD	371	0.4	3.9	39.3	0.3
Garlic & Herb Reduced Calorie Salad Dressing HELLMANN'S	233	0.7	13.1	19.3	0.4
Herb 'n' Garlic Dressing, Light KRAFT	116	1.3	15.5	5.1	0.2
Honey & Mustard Dressing, Light KRAFT	131	1.3	19	5	1.2
Italian Dressing					
Classic KRAFT	120	0.1	5.6	10.3	0.3
Light KRAFT	32	0.1	6.8	Tr	0.6
low carbohydrate CARB OPTIONS	233	0.2	0.8	25.3	0.8
low fat, Waistline					
CROSSE & BLACKWELL	110	0.8	11.9	6.6	n/a
luxury HELLMANN'S	269	0.5	19.5	20.8	0.3
warm HELLMANN'S	411	2.1	13.9	38.5	1
Low Fat Dressing WEIGHT WATCHERS	107	1.4	16	4.2	0
Classic light HELLMANN'S	61	0.4	9.5	2.7	1.2

All amounts per 100g/100ml unless otherwise stated	Cal kcal	Pro g	Carb g	Fat g	Fibre g
Mayonnaise	**691**	1.1	1.7	75.6	0
HEINZ	**734**	1.5	0.4	80.7	0
extra light HELLMANN'S	**106**	0.5	11.3	6.4	0.2
light CARB OPTION	**288**	0.7	4.6	29.8	Tr
light WEIGHT WATCHERS	**280**	1	7.3	27.7	0.7
light, reduced calorie HELLMANN'S	**299**	0.7	6.7	29.8	Tr
organic MERIDIAN FOODS LTD	**660**	0.9	3.6	71.3	n/a
Real BURGESS	**717**	1.4	3	77.5	0.4
Real HELLMANN'S	**722**	1.1	1.3	79.1	0
Salad BURGESS	**579**	2.4	8.1	59.2	0
Mustard, Mild, Low Fat Dressing					
WEIGHT WATCHERS	**63**	2	5.7	3.6	0
Carb Check HEINZ	**69**	1.9	5.5	3.7	Tr
Miracle Whip Dressing KRAFT	**380**	0.3	12.5	36	0.1
Salad Cream	**348**	1.5	16.7	31	N
HEINZ	**331**	1.4	20.3	26.7	Tr
light HEINZ	**244**	1.8	13.5	19.9	Tr
low fat, Waistline					
CROSSE & BLACKWELL	**5**	0.3	0.4	0.2	n/a
organic MERIDIAN FOODS LTD	**346**	1.9	11.6	32.1	0.2
reduced calorie	**194**	1	9.4	17.2	
Seafood Sauce BAXTERS	**532**	1.9	9.7	53.9	0.7
COLMAN'S	**296**	0.9	21.7	22.9	0.5
Tandoori Warm Dressing					
HELLMANN'S	**397**	1.9	13.8	37.1	1

All amounts per 100g/100ml unless otherwise stated	Cal kcal	Pro g	Carb g	Fat g	Fibre g
Thai Warm Dressing HELLMANN'S	**406**	1.7	16.7	36.9	0.8
Thousand Island Dressing					
HELLMANN'S	**197**	0.4	13.7	15.6	0.3
Classic KRAFT	**365**	0.9	19.5	31.5	0.4
fat free KRAFT	**90**	0.5	20.5	0.2	2.8
low carbohydrate CARB OPTIONS	**158**	0.6	3.9	15.6	1.2
Vinaigrette light HELLMANN'S	**49**	Tr	12.2	Tr	0.2
light, Waistline CROSSE & BLACKWELL	**5**	0.3	0.4	0.2	n/a

CHUTNEYS & PICKLES

Albert's Victorian Chutney BAXTERS	**153**	0.9	36.2	0.4	n/a
Apple Chutney	**190**	0.9	49.2	0.2	n/a
Apple & Onion Sweet Chutney GARNER'S	**179**	0.6	44	0.1	1
Beetroot Pickle, Spreadable HAYWARD'S	**79**	1.1	18.3	0.1	n/a
Barbecue Relish BICK'S	**93**	1.8	21.1	0.2	n/a
Branston Original CROSSE & BLACKWELL	**109**	0.8	26.1	0.2	n/a
Branston Smooth Pickle CROSSE & BLACKWELL	**125**	0.9	29.8	0.2	n/a
Cabbage, Pickled GARNER'S	**65**	0.9	14.9	0.2	1.1

All amounts per 100g/100ml unless otherwise stated	Cal kcal	Pro g	Carb g	Fat g	Fibre g
Caramelised Red Onion Chutney LOYD GROSSMAN	**223**	1.2	54	0.2	n/a
Chilli Pickle PATAK	**325**	4.3	1.3	33.7	0
Crushed Pineapple & Sweet Pepper Chutney BAXTERS	**163**	1.1	28	5.2	n/a
Cranberry & Caramelised Red Onion Chutney BAXTERS	**154**	0.3	38	0.1	n/a
Eggs, Pickled GARNER'S	**83**	7.1	0.3	5.9	0
Gherkins, pickled	**14**	0.9	2.6	0.1	n/a
pickled GARNER'S	**38**	0.5	8.8	0.1	0.7
sliced, dill HAYWARD'S	**34**	1	5.5	0.5	n/a
whole HAYWARD'S	**34**	1	5.5	0.5	n/a
Hot Mango Pickle PATAK	**270**	2.3	7.4	25.7	1.9
Lime Pickle, Medium Hot PATAK	**194**	2.2	4	18.7	0.4
Mango & Apricot Chutney LOYD GROSSMAN	**214**	1.2	51.8	0.2	n/a
Mango Chutney					
BAXTERS	**173**	0.5	42	0.3	n/a
GARNER'S	**203**	0.5	50	0.1	1.5
Bengal Spice SHARWOOD	**243**	0.3	60.1	0.1	1.8
Green Label SHARWOOD	**241**	0.3	59.7	0.1	1.1
Major Grey Sweet SHARWOOD	**240**	0.2	59.6	Tr	1.2
Tropical Lime SHARWOOD	**240**	0.3	57.6	0.9	1.7

All amounts per 100g/100ml unless otherwise stated	Cal kcal	Pro g	Carb g	Fat g	Fibre g
Mustard Pickle, mild					
HEINZ	**129**	2.2	25.7	1.3	0.9
Branston CROSSE & BLACKWELL	**108**	0.9	24.7	0.6	n/a
Onion Pickle GARNER'S	**163**	0.5	40	0.1	0.6
Onions, pickled drained	**35**	0.8	7	0.5	1
GARNER'S	**55**	0.8	12.8	0.1	0.8
HAYWARD'S	**23**	0.7	4.7	0.1	n/a
organic HAYWARD'S	**31**	0.8	6.7	0	n/a
silverskin GARNER'S	**85**	0.8	20.3	0.1	0.8
silverskin HAYWARD'S	**10**	0.4	1.9	0.1	n/a
Piccalilli GARNER'S	**108**	2	23	0.9	0.8
HAYWARD'S	**66**	1.4	13.9	0.5	n/a
HEINZ	**107**	1.7	21.6	0.7	0.6
spreadable sweet HAYWARD'S	**105**	1.2	24.4	0.3	n/a
wholegrain & Dijon Mustard,					
Branston CROSSE & BLACKWELL	**75**	1.3	15.8	0.7	n/a
Ploughman's Pickle HEINZ	**117**	0.8	26.7	0.2	0.9
Sandwich Pickle, tangy HEINZ	**134**	0.7	31.4	0.2	0.9
Branston CROSSE & BLACKWELL	**109**	0.8	26.1	0.2	n/a
Sauerkraut	**9**	1.1	1.1	Tr	n/a
Shallots, pickled GARNER'S	**76**	0.9	17.9	0.1	0.7
Spanish Tomato & Black Olive Chutney BAXTERS	**133**	1.8	29	1.1	n/a
Spiced Cranberry Chutney LOYD GROSSMAN	**176**	0.7	43.1	0.1	n/a

All amounts per 100g/100ml unless otherwise stated	Cal kcal	Pro g	Carb g	Fat g	Fibre g
Spiced Fruit Chutney BAXTERS	145	0.6	34.9	0.3	n/a
Spreadable Chutney, Green Label SHARWOOD	241	0.3	59.7	0.1	1.1
Sweet Pickle	141	0.6	36	0.1	n/a
Sweet Tomato Chutney LOYD GROSSMAN	145	1.7	34.2	0.2	n/a
Traditional Pickle, Spreadable HAYWARD'S	149	1	35.8	0.2	n/a
Tomato Chutney	128	1.2	31	0.2	n/a
BAXTERS	158	1.7	37.1	0.3	n/a
Tomato Pickle, tangy HEINZ	106	2	22	0.3	1.5

COOKING SAUCES & MARINADES

All amounts per 100g/100ml unless otherwise stated	Cal kcal	Pro g	Carb g	Fat g	Fibre g
TRADITIONAL					
Ale & Mushroom Beef Tonight Sauce KNORR	**58**	0.8	6.3	3.3	0.2
Basic Tomato Cook-In-Sauce HOMEPRIDE	**52**	0.9	7.1	2.2	0.7
Bechamel Sauce LOYD GROSSMAN	**105**	0.7	6.1	8.6	n/a
Bechamel Sauce Mix, Bonne Cuisine, as prepared CROSSE & BLACKWELL	**73**	3.7	9.7	2.2	0.5
Beef & Ale Dry Casserole Mix, as sold COLMAN'S	**320**	9.2	66.3	2	2.3
Beef Casserole Dry Casserole Mix, as sold COLMAN'S	**308**	7.5	66	1.5	2.5
Bourguignon Beef Tonight Sauce KNORR	**57**	0.6	7.6	2.6	0.4
Bread Sauce					
made with semi-skimmed milk	**97**	4.2	15.3	2.5	n/a
made with whole milk	**110**	4.1	15.2	4	n/a
Bread Sauce Mix, as sold COLMAN'S	**327**	11.4	67.9	1.1	3.2
Classic Dry Sauce Mix KNORR	**356**	10.8	60	8.1	3
Chicken Casserole Mix, as sold SCHWARTZ	**363**	10.4	70.7	4.3	2

All amounts per 100g/100ml unless otherwise stated	Cal kcal	Pro g	Carb g	Fat g	Fibre g
Cheddar Cheese Dry Sauce Mix,					
as sold COLMAN'S	**407**	18.3	48.8	15.4	1.2
Mature Dry Sauce Mix KNORR	**457**	19	39.1	25	2.3
Cheese & Bacon Pasta Bake Sauce					
HOMEPRIDE	**84**	2.7	5.1	5.9	0.5
Cheese Sauce, recipe					
made with semi-skimmed milk	**181**	8.2	8.8	12.8	n/a
made with whole milk	**198**	8.1	8.7	14.8	n/a
Cheese Sauce Packet Mix					
made with semi-skimmed milk	**91**	5.5	9.2	3.8	N
made with whole milk	**111**	5.4	9	6	N
Cheddar Cheese Sauce					
Mix, as sold SCHWARTZ	**363**	16.9	61.6	5.5	2.1
Cheese Sauce Granules, as sold					
BISTO	**482**	6.9	51.1	27.8	1.2
Chicken Supreme Cook-In-Sauce					
HOMEPRIDE	**122**	0.7	3.8	11.5	0.6
Chicken Supreme Dry Casserole					
Mix, as sold COLMAN'S	**358**	12.1	56.7	9.2	2.4
Classic White Sauce Dry Mix,					
as sold COLMAN'S	**335**	10.7	66.5	2.9	2.6
Coronation Sauce HEINZ	**334**	0.8	13.1	31	0.9
Cracked Peppercorn & Cream Pour					
Over Sauce, as sold KNORR	**145**	1	3.3	14.2	0.4

All amounts per 100g/100ml unless otherwise stated	Cal kcal	Pro g	Carb g	Fat g	Fibre g
Creamy Cheese & Bacon Pasta Bake Dry Casserole Mix, as sold COLMAN'S	**359**	17	54.8	8	1.8
Creamy Ham & Mushroom Pasta Stir Sauce HOMEPRIDE	**123**	2.6	4.3	10.7	0.4
Creamy Mushroom Chicken Tonight Sauce KNORR	**88**	0.4	4.3	7.7	0.3
low fat	**48**	0.3	5.3	2.9	0.4
Creamy Mushroom Sauce CARB OPTIONS	**76**	0.7	3.5	6.6	0.4
Creamy Parsley with Lemon Pour Over Sauce, as sold KNORR	**153**	0.8	3.8	14.9	0.6
Creamy Pepper Pourover Dry Sauce Mix, as sold KNORR	**327**	9.1	65.3	3.2	2
Creamy Pepper & Mushroom Dry Sauce Mix, as sold COLMAN'S	**332**	9.6	64.6	3.8	3
Creamy Tomato & Bacon Pasta Bake Sauce HOMEPRIDE	**95**	2	7	6.5	0.7
Creamy Tomato & Herb Pasta Bake Sauce HOMEPRIDE	**104**	1.6	8.2	7.2	0.9
Creamy Tomato Pasta Bake Dry Casserole Mix, as sold COLMAN'S	**315**	10.8	60.7	3.2	5
Four Cheese Dry Sauce Mix, as sold COLMAN'S	**362**	17.1	48.4	11.1	1.8

All amounts per 100g/100ml unless otherwise stated	Cal kcal	Pro g	Carb g	Fat g	Fibre g
Four Cheese Pasta Bake Sauce					
HOMEPRIDE	85	2.7	4.2	6.4	0.4
Hearty Cumberland Sausages					
Tonight Sauce KNORR	33	0.7	7.4	0.1	0.8
Hollandaise Dry Sauce Mix,					
as sold COLMAN'S	372	6.4	61.6	11.1	1.8
Hollandaise Sauce					
Bonne Cuisine Mix, as sold					
CROSSE & BLACKWELL	390	10	50.3	16.8	1.6
pour over sauce, as sold KNORR	202	0.6	3.9	20.5	0.4
Honey & Mustard Chicken					
Tonight Sauce KNORR	109	1	14.2	5.4	0.8
low fat	80	1	13.8	2.3	0.8
Honey & Mustard Cook-In-Sauce					
HOMEPRIDE	86	0.9	14.3	2.8	0.4
Honey Chicken Dry Casserole					
Mix, as sold COLMAN'S	341	2.6	80.2	1.1	0.6
Hot Pot Cook-In-Sauce					
HOMEPRIDE	33	0.6	7.5	0.1	0.6
Lamb Hotpot Dry Casserole					
Mix, as sold COLMAN'S	297	6.9	63.3	1.7	2.1
Lamb Ragout Classic Creations					
Mix, as sold CROSSE & BLACKWELL	340	9.5	59.9	6.9	1.9

All amounts per 100g/100ml unless otherwise stated	Cal kcal	Pro g	Carb g	Fat g	Fibre g
Ginger Marinade LEA & PERRINS	**116**	0.3	28.8	Tr	0.9
Liver & Bacon Dry Casserole Mix, as sold COLMAN'S	**303**	10.3	61.6	1.7	4.7
Luxury Peppercorn Pourover Dry Sauce Mix, as sold KNORR	**307**	9.7	65.3	0.8	1.7
Madeira Wine Gravy Sauce Mix, Bonne Cuisine, as prepared CROSSE & BLACKWELL	**40**	0.9	7.8	0.6	0.4
Mushroom & Garlic Cook-In-Sauce HOMEPRIDE	**81**	0.8	6	6	0.3
Onion Sauce made with semi-skimmed milk	**88**	3	8.2	5.1	n/a
made with whole milk	**101**	2.9	8.1	6.6	n/a
Onion Dry Sauce Mix, as sold COLMAN'S	**325**	10.7	66.5	2.9	2.6
Parsley Dry Sauce Mix, as sold COLMAN'S	**314**	7.2	67.9	1.5	3.7
Parsley Sauce Mix, Creamy, as sold SCHWARTZ	**402**	10.6	58.9	13.7	2.3
Pepper Sauce Mix, Creamy, as sold SCHWARTZ	**349**	17.9	56.8	5.5	3.5
Pork Dry Casserole Mix, as sold COLMAN'S	**328**	6.7	72	1.4	2.8

All amounts per 100g/100ml unless otherwise stated	Cal kcal	Pro g	Carb g	Fat g	Fibre g
Potato Bake Cheddar Mix					
BATCHELORS	**386**	11.4	46.7	17	8.3
Potato Bake Cheese & Onion Mix					
BATCHELORS	**360**	9.6	48	14.4	9.7
Prawn Cocktail Sauce BURGESS	**336**	2.3	20.1	26.6	0.8
Red Wine & Herbs RAGU	**37**	1.3	7.6	0.1	0.9
Red Wine Cook-In-Sauce					
HOMEPRIDE	**46**	0.4	9.8	0.6	0.3
Rich Red Wine & Onion Sausages Tonight Sauce KNORR	**35**	0.5	7.8	0.2	0.6
Rich Sausage & Onion Dry Casserole Mix, as sold COLMAN'S	**318**	9.6	64.2	2.6	2.6
Rich Tomato Beef Tonight Sauce					
KNORR	**50**	1.7	8.3	1.1	1.1
Roaster Garlic & Herb Coating Mix BATCHELORS	**316**	9.5	47.1	11.4	7.8
Sauce de Paris Mix, Bonne Cuisine, as sold CROSSE & BLACKWELL	**335**	11.6	48.6	10.1	2.4
Sausage & Tomato Classic Creations Mix, as sold CROSSE & BLACKWELL	**375**	11.7	61.1	8.4	2.4
Sausage Casserole Cook-In-Sauce					
HOMEPRIDE	**37**	0.7	8	0.2	0.6

All amounts per 100g/100ml unless otherwise stated	Cal kcal	Pro g	Carb g	Fat g	Fibre g
Shepherd's Pie Classic Creations					
Mix, as sold CROSSE & BLACKWELL	**300**	12.1	48	6.2	1.6
Shepherd's Pie Cook-In-Sauce					
HOMEPRIDE	**40**	1.2	8.1	0.3	1
Shepherd's Pie Dry Casserole					
Mix, as sold COLMAN'S	**282**	12.5	54.7	1.4	4.3
Toad in the Hole Dry Casserole					
Mix, as sold COLMAN'S	**336**	17.7	64.2	0.9	2.5
Tomato & Herb Marinade					
LEA & PERRINS	**107**	1	26	0.3	1
Tomato, Onion & Garlic					
Pasta Stir HOMEPRIDE	**56**	0.8	8.2	2.2	0.6
Traditional Chicken Dry					
Casserole Mix, as sold COLMAN'S	**311**	5.7	69.4	0.1	1.5
Traditional Sausage Dry					
Casserole Mix, as sold COLMAN'S	**324**	9.3	68.9	1.2	4.4
Tuna Pasta Bake Dry					
Casserole Mix, as sold COLMAN'S	**331**	10.4	60.5	5.3	4.4
Turkey Casserole Dry					
Casserole Mix, as sold COLMAN'S	**313**	5.9	68	1.9	3.5
White Sauce, savoury, recipe					
made with semi-skimmed milk	**130**	4.4	10.7	8	n/a
made with whole milk	**151**	4.2	10.6	10.3	n/a

All amounts per 100g/100ml unless otherwise stated	Cal kcal	Pro g	Carb g	Fat g	Fibre g
White Sauce Granules, as sold					
BISTO	**480**	3.3	54.1	27.9	2.5
White Sauce Mix, savoury,					
as sold COLMAN'S	**335**	10.7	66.5	2.9	2.6
White Wine & Cream					
Cook-in-Sauce HOMEPRIDE	**76**	1.1	7.8	4.5	0.2
White Wine Gravy Sauce Mix,					
Bonne Cuisine, as sold					
CROSSE & BLACKWELL	**350**	7.8	66.7	5.6	1.2

CHINESE

Black Bean & Red Pepper					
Cooking Sauce SHARWOOD	**62**	1.9	10.5	1.4	1.2
Black Bean Stir Fry Creations,					
as sold CROSSE & BLACKWELL	**375**	10.8	65.3	7.6	2.8
Black Bean Stir Fry Sauce AMOY	**152**	3.8	33.7	0.2	n/a
SHARWOOD	**98**	2.2	18.8	1.5	0.6
Black Bean with Green					
Pepper Sauce UNCLE BEN'S	**70**	1.9	12.7	1.3	n/a
Cantonese Sauce UNCLE BEN'S	**105**	0.6	25.5	Tr	n/a
Just for One UNCLE BEN'S	**101**	0.6	24.5	Tr	n/a
Chilli & Garlic Sauce					
LEA & PERRINS	**60**	1	14.9	n/a	n/a

All amounts per 100g/100ml unless otherwise stated	Cal kcal	Pro g	Carb g	Fat g	Fibre g
Chinese 5 Spice Stir it Up KNORR	632	3	35.8	53	2.7
Chinese BBQ & Sesame Coating Sauce SHARWOOD	66	0.6	12.1	1.7	1.2
Chinese Szechuan Cooking Sauce WEIGHT WATCHERS	48	1.2	7.7	1.4	0.8
Chow Mein Mix ROSS	58	2.2	13.3	0.4	1.8
Chow Mein Stir Fry Sauce BLUE DRAGON	92	1.1	15.4	2.9	0.4
Cracked Black Pepper Stir Fry Sauce AMOY	256	1.8	51	5	n/a
Hoi Sin & Plum Cooking Sauce SHARWOOD	94	0.7	19.9	1.3	0.9
Hoi Sin & Spring Onion Stir-Fry Sauce SHARWOOD	119	1.3	26.5	0.9	0.8
Hoi Sin Sauce for Spare Ribs SHARWOOD	149	1.5	33.3	0.5	1.3
Hoi Sin Sauce with Spring Onion UNCLE BEN'S	104	1.1	18.9	2.7	n/a
Honey & Coriander Stir Fry Sauce BLUE DRAGON	96	0.5	22.1	0.6	0.3
Hong Kong Curry Oriental Sauces LOYD GROSSMAN	106	1.3	7.8	7.7	n/a

All amounts per 100g/100ml unless otherwise stated	Cal kcal	Pro g	Carb g	Fat g	Fibre g
Lemon & Sesame Stir-Fry Sauce SHARWOOD	125	0.1	30.9	0.1	0.1
Lemon Chicken Sauce UNCLE BEN'S	100	0.3	24	0.3	n/a
Light Soy Sauce SHARWOOD	37	2.7	6.4	0.2	Tr
Oriental Beef Stir Fry Creations, as sold CROSSE & BLACKWELL	350	9	66	5.3	1.1
Oriental Chicken Stir Fry Creations, as sold CROSSE & BLACKWELL	335	6.1	70.9	2.8	0.4
Oriental Sweet & Sour Cooking Sauce WEIGHT WATCHERS	51	0.8	11.7	0.1	0.8
Oyster & Garlic Stir Fry Sauce, Rich AMOY	151	3.1	33.5	0.5	n/a
Plum Sauce SHARWOOD	240	0.2	59.5	0.1	1
Stir Fry AMOY	255	0.2	62.6	0.4	n/a
Oyster & Mushroom Cooking Sauce SHARWOOD	60	0.7	10.2	1.8	1.6
Oyster Sauce SHARWOOD	67	2.7	13.6	0.2	Tr
Peking Lemon Stir Fry Sauce BLUE DRAGON	166	0.3	36.8	1.9	0.1
Rich Soy Sauce SHARWOOD	79	3.1	16.6	0.4	Tr
Spicy Tomato Szechuan Stir-Fry Sauce SHARWOOD	79	1.3	17.5	0.3	0.8

All amounts per 100g/100ml unless otherwise stated	Cal kcal	Pro g	Carb g	Fat g	Fibre g
Sweet & Sour Barbecue Sauce					
HEINZ	**125**	1	26.3	1.7	0.4
Sweet & Sour Chicken Tonight					
Sauce KNORR	**85**	0.4	20.8	0.1	0.5
Sweet & Sour Cooking Sauce					
SHARWOOD	**105**	0.6	24.5	0.5	0.8
Sweet & Sour Cook-In-Sauce					
HOMEPRIDE	**98**	0.4	23.9	0.1	0.5
Sweet & Sour Sauce					
UNCLE BEN'S	**86**	0.5	20.9	0.1	n/a
Just for One UNCLE BEN'S	**130**	0.7	27.5	1.9	n/a
light UNCLE BEN'S	**60**	0.6	14.2	Tr	n/a
Oriental Sauces LOYD GROSSMAN	**136**	1.2	28	2.1	n/a
Stir Fry AMOY	**221**	0.5	54.4	0.2	n/a
with extra pineapple UNCLE BEN'S	**88**	0.5	21.4	0.1	n/a
Sweet & Sour Stir-Fry Sauce					
SHARWOOD	**112**	0.5	27.2	0.1	Tr
Sweet 'n' Sour Dry Sauce Mix,					
as sold COLMAN'S	**337**	2.3	81	0.5	1.4
Sweet & Sour Sizzle & Stir KNORR	**151**	0.5	16.7	9.1	1
Sweet Chilli & Lemongrass					
Stir-Fry Sauce SHARWOOD	**82**	0.3	19.7	0.1	0.3
Sweet Chilli Cooking Sauce					
SHARWOOD	**70**	0.6	16.6	0.1	1.1

All amounts per 100g/100ml unless otherwise stated	Cal kcal	Pro g	Carb g	Fat g	Fibre g
Sweet Chilli Sauce SHARWOOD	**182**	0.7	43.7	0.3	0.1
Szechuan Spicy Tomato Stir Fry Sauce BLUE DRAGON	**126**	1.3	17.6	5.6	2
Wok Soy Sauce SHARWOOD	**139**	5.6	26.7	11	0.2
Yellow Bean Sauce AMOY	**155**	3.3	33.1	1	n/a
Yellow Bean Stir Fry Sauce SHARWOOD	**104**	1.1	23.5	0.6	0.1

ITALIAN

All amounts per 100g/100ml unless otherwise stated	Cal kcal	Pro g	Carb g	Fat g	Fibre g
Basil & Oregano Sauce RAGU	**37**	1.4	7.7	0.1	1
Bolognese Express Pasta Sauce DOLMIO	**88**	7.4	7.1	3.3	n/a
Bolognese Sauce					
recipe	**161**	11.8	2.5	11.6	n/a
LOYD GROSSMAN	**68**	2.1	8.7	2.8	n/a
Carb Check HEINZ	**53**	3.8	3.6	2.6	0.4
original DOLMIO	**52**	1.7	8.7	1.2	n/a
original RAGU	**37**	1.4	7.6	0.1	0.9
original, light DOLMIO	**39**	1.6	8	0.1	n/a
Bolognese Extra Onion & Garlic Express Pasta Sauce DOLMIO	**89**	7.4	7.3	3.3	n/a
Bolognese with Extra Mushroom Express Pasta Sauce DOLMIO	**91**	7.8	7.4	3.3	n/a

All amounts per 100g/100ml unless otherwise stated	Cal kcal	Pro g	Carb g	Fat g	Fibre g
Carbonara Pasta Sauce					
LOYD GROSSMAN	**127**	3.5	7.5	9.1	n/a
NAPOLINA	**150**	3.9	4.8	12.8	n/a
Chargrilled Vegetable Sauce, as sold BERTOLLI	**53**	2	6.9	2	1.3
Chunky Sweet Pepper Bolognese Sauce DOLMIO	**54**	1.3	9	1.4	n/a
Chunky Mediterranean Vegetables Bolognese Sauce DOLMIO	**55**	1.3	8.8	1.6	n/a
Chunky Mushroom & Courgette Bolognese Sauce DOLMIO	**53**	1.5	8.5	1.5	n/a
Chunky Roasted Onion & Garlic Bolognese Sauce DOLMIO	**56**	1.5	8.7	1.6	n/a
Creamy Carbonara Express Pasta Sauce DOLMIO	**149**	3.4	4.2	13.2	n/a
Creamy Carbonara Stir-in Sauce DOLMIO	**181**	5.5	4.3	15.8	n/a
Creamy Ham & Mushroom Pasta Stir HOMEPRIDE	**123**	2.6	4.3	10.7	0.4
Creamy Mushroom Express Pasta Sauce DOLMIO	**107**	1.4	3.8	9.6	n/a
Creamy Mushroom Pasta Bake DOLMIO	**105**	1.3	5.7	8.6	n/a

All amounts per 100g/100ml unless otherwise stated	Cal kcal	Pro g	Carb g	Fat g	Fibre g
Creamy Tomato & Cheese Pasta Bake DOLMIO	**55**	2.2	8.8	1.2	n/a
Creamy Tomato Pasta Bake DOLMIO	**102**	1.5	8.7	6.8	n/a
Creamy Tomato Pasta Sauce, Carb Check HEINZ	**61**	2	4.2	4	0.5
Creamy Tomato Sauce, Waistline CROSSE & BLACKWELL	**89**	2.7	14.4	2.3	n/a
Extra Onion & Garlic Bolognese Sauce DOLMIO	**53**	1.7	9	1	n/a
Extra Mushrooms Bolognese Sauce DOLMIO	**50**	1.7	8.4	1.1	n/a
Extra Spicy Bolognese Sauce DOLMIO	**52**	1.7	8.8	1.1	n/a
Italian Pasta Cooking Sauce WEIGHT WATCHERS	**38**	1.5	7.6	0.2	0.9
Italian Spicy Chilli Stir-in Sauce DOLMIO	**140**	1.5	9.3	10.7	n/a
Italian Tomato Pasta Sauces GO ORGANIC					
and aubergine	**67**	1.2	3.9	5.2	1
and black olive	**68**	1.1	3.6	5.5	0.9
and red chilli	**75**	1.3	5	5.5	1.2
and sweet basil	**64**	1.2	4.3	4.7	0.9
and sweet pepper	**77**	1.3	5.8	5.4	1.2

All amounts per 100g/100ml unless otherwise stated	Cal kcal	Pro g	Carb g	Fat g	Fibre g
Italian Tomato with Sun-Ripened Tomato & Basil UNCLE BEN'S	41.5	1	7.8	0.6	0.6
Italienne Tomato & Herbs Stir it Up KNORR	649	5.6	18.2	61.5	2.5
Lasagne Creamy Pasta Bake NAPOLINA	85	2.9	9.4	4	0.1
Mediterranean Vegetable Sauce, as sold BERTOLLI	88	1.7	4.1	7.2	0.7
Mushroom, Garlic, Oregano & Tomato Sauce, as sold BERTOLLI	90	1.9	3.8	7.5	0.9
Mushroom Sauce, organic MERIDIAN FOODS LTD	65	1.8	8	2.8	1
Olive Sauce, organic MERIDIAN FOODS LTD	64	1.5	7.3	3.2	1.1
Onion & Garlic Sauce RAGU	37	1.4	7.7	0.1	0.9
Pasta 'n' Sauce BATCHELORS					
bolognese	353	15.1	67.2	2.6	3.9
carbonara	386	14.3	71	5	3.1
cheese, leek & ham	378	16.1	67	5.1	2
chicken & mushroom	361	14.1	72.3	1.7	2.8
chicken & roasted garlic	372	12.6	73.8	2.9	3.4
macaroni cheese	372	17.2	65.2	4.7	2.7
mild cheese & broccoli	363	15	67	3.9	4
mushroom & wine	377	12	71.3	4.9	2.5
tomato, onion & herbs	348	13.8	68.8	2	4

All amounts per 100g/100ml unless otherwise stated	Cal kcal	Pro g	Carb g	Fat g	Fibre g
Pasta Sauce, tomato based	**47**	2	6.9	1.5	N
Piccanti Pasta Sauce LOYD GROSSMAN	**92**	1.5	8	6	n/a
Primavera Pasta Sauce LOYD GROSSMAN	**98**	1.4	6.3	7.4	n/a
Puttanesca Pasta Sauce LOYD GROSSMAN	**90**	1.7	6.8	6.2	n/a
Red Pepper & Chilli, organic MERIDIAN FOODS LTD	**99**	1.5	10.6	5.5	1.1
Rich Tomato with Basil Pesto Express Pasta Sauce DOLMIO	**86**	2	6.2	5.9	n/a
Roasted Vegetable Express Pasta Sauce DOLMIO	**51**	1.4	7.5	1.7	n/a
Roasted Vegetables Stir-in Sauce DOLMIO	**134**	1.5	8.7	10.3	n/a
Slow Roasted Garlic & Tomato Stir-in Sauce DOLMIO	**136**	1.6	9.8	10	n/a
Smokey Bacon & Tomato Stir-in Sauce DOLMIO	**165**	5.5	6.9	12.8	n/a
Smoky Bacon Pasta Sauce LOYD GROSSMAN	**98**	3.1	5.4	7.2	n/a
Spaghetti Bolognese Classic Creations Mix, as sold CROSSE & BLACKWELL	**275**	11.4	42.1	6.3	2.7

All amounts per 100g/100ml unless otherwise stated	Cal kcal	Pro g	Carb g	Fat g	Fibre g
Spaghetti Bolognese with Mushrooms Dry Casserole Mix, as sold COLMAN'S	307	7.8	66.8	0.9	4.7
Spicy Arrabbiata Premium Pasta Sauce NAPOLINA	62	1.3	7.2	3.1	0.9
Spicy Bolognese Sauce RAGU	37	1.4	7.6	0.1	0.9
Spicy Italian Chilli Express Pasta Sauce DOLMIO	51	1.5	7.5	1.6	n/a
Spicy Pepperoni & Tomato Stir-in Sauce DOLMIO	154	3.2	9.3	11.6	n/a
Spicy Tomato & Pepperoni Pasta Bake Sauce HOMEPRIDE	74	1.6	8.6	3.7	0.9
Sun-Dried Tomato Pasta Stir HOMEPRIDE	64	1.1	7.4	3.3	0.8
Sun-Dried Tomato Stir-in Sauce DOLMIO	153	1.7	11.1	11.3	n/a
light	92	1.7	10.7	4.7	n/a
Sun-Ripened Tomato & Basil Express Pasta Sauce DOLMIO	52	1.5	7.9	1.6	n/a
Sweet Chilli, Red Onion & Tomato Sauce, as sold BERTOLLI	91	1.7	4.9	7.2	0.7
Sweet Pepper Stir-in Sauce DOLMIO	137	1.5	9.7	10.3	n/a

All amounts per 100g/100ml unless otherwise stated	Cal kcal	Pro g	Carb g	Fat g	Fibre g
Sweet Pepper & Tomato Sauce,					
as sold BERTOLLI	**89**	1.5	4.3	7.2	0.5
Sweet Red Pepper Pasta Sauce					
LOYD GROSSMAN	**87**	1.7	7.3	5.6	n/a
Tomato & Bacon Pasta Stir					
HOMEPRIDE	**86**	2.6	8.5	4.6	0.8
Tomato & Balsamic Vinegar Pasta Sauce LOYD GROSSMAN	**93**	1.6	8.3	5.9	n/a
Tomato & Basil Pasta Stir					
HOMEPRIDE	**57**	1.1	6.4	3	0.8
Tomato & Basil Sauce,					
as sold BERTOLLI	**50**	1.9	8.6	0.9	1.2
as sold LOYD GROSSMAN	**90**	1.7	7.9	5.7	n/a
Carb Check HEINZ	**56**	1.5	4.4	3.6	0.6
Waistline CROSSE & BLACKWELL	**68**	2.4	11.9	1.2	n/a
Tomato & Chargrilled Courgette Pasta Sauce LOYD GROSSMAN	**83**	1.4	6.8	5.6	n/a
Tomato & Chargrilled Vegetable Pasta Sauce LOYD GROSSMAN	**89**	1.8	7.9	5.6	n/a
Tomato & Chilli Pasta Sauce					
LOYD GROSSMAN	**88**	1.7	7.3	5.7	n/a
Tomato & Garlic Pasta Sauce					
LOYD GROSSMAN	**92**	2	8.8	5.5	n/a

All amounts per 100g/100ml unless otherwise stated	Cal kcal	Pro g	Carb g	Fat g	Fibre g
Tomato & Marscarpone Pasta					
Sauce LOYD GROSSMAN	**138**	2.3	9	10.4	n/a
NAPOLINA	**95**	1.5	4.8	8	n/a
Tomato & Mushroom					
Pasta Sauce LOYD GROSSMAN	**88**	2.1	7.4	5.6	n/a
Tomato, Basil & Green Pesto					
Pasta Sauce NAPOLINA	**85**	1.3	5.6	6.5	n/a
Tomato, Chilli & Garlic Pasta					
Sauce NAPOLINA	**80**	1.7	6.4	5.5	n/a
Tomato Lasagne Sauce DOLMIO	**52**	1.7	8.8	1.1	n/a
RAGU	**39**	1.2	8.4	0.1	0.8
Tomato, Red Wine & Shallots					
Sauce, as sold BERTOLLI	**49**	2	6.1	1.9	1.2
Tomato, Roasted Garlic &					
Mushroom Sauce, as sold					
BERTOLLI	**47**	1.9	5.3	1.9	1.2
Tomato, Romano & Garlic Sauce,					
as sold BERTOLLI	**66**	2.5	7.2	3.1	1.2
Tomato Sauce CARB OPTIONS	**26**	1.4	5	0.1	0.9
Tomato/Herb Sauce, organic					
MERIDIAN FOODS LTD	**64**	1.6	8.1	2.8	1.1
Traditional Sauce for Bolognese					
RAGU	**45**	1.6	5.8	1.8	0.1

All amounts per 100g/100ml unless otherwise stated	Cal kcal	Pro g	Carb g	Fat g	Fibre g
White Lasagne Sauce DOLMIO	**96**	0.6	7	7.3	n/a
RAGU	**158**	0.6	4.8	15.2	0.3

INDIAN

Achari Cooking Sauce					
SHARWOOD	**171**	3.9	18.1	9.2	2.4
Balti Cooking Sauce					
LOYD GROSSMAN	**163**	1.7	8.8	13.4	n/a
SHARWOOD	**80**	1.5	8.2	4.6	3.2
Balti Sizzle & Stir KNORR	**118**	1	6.7	9.7	0.7
Beer & Mushroom Balti Cooking Sauce PATAK	**107**	1.4	7.1	7.1	0.9
Bhuna Cooking Sauce					
LOYD GROSSMAN	**144**	2.6	11.6	9.7	n/a
SHARWOOD	**111**	1.3	11.3	6.8	2.3
Chicken Curry Indian Creations Mix, as sold CROSSE & BLACKWELL	**305**	8.1	50.1	7.3	4.8
Chicken Korma Dry Casserole Mix, as sold COLMAN'S	**448**	7	44	27.1	8.6
Chip Shop Curry Sauce Dry Mix, as sold COLMAN'S	**342**	3.6	78.8	1.4	2.4
Creamy Curry Chicken Tonight Sauce KNORR	**78**	0.6	2.3	7.4	0.8

All amounts per 100g/100ml unless otherwise stated	Cal kcal	Pro g	Carb g	Fat g	Fibre g
Curry Cook-In-Sauce HOMEPRIDE	56	1.1	8.6	1.9	0.5
Curry Powder SHARWOOD					
hot	247	14.1	17.9	13.2	32.1
medium	210	12.4	11.1	12.9	41.1
mild	228	15	16.2	11.5	35.5
Curry Paste					
Balti with Tomato & Coriander					
PATAK	391	4.1	17.2	34	2.2
Garam Masala PATAK	403	3.2	17.9	35.4	0.6
Korma PATAK	535	4.2	13	51.8	2.6
Korma SHARWOOD	352	4.1	9.5	33.1	9.9
Madras SHARWOOD	436	2.5	11.8	42	13.4
Madras, hot PATAK	586	4.3	21.6	53.6	5.2
Rogan Josh PATAK	397	4.1	12.7	36.7	5.9
Rogan Josh SHARWOOD	398	5.2	9.1	37.9	11.7
Tandoori PATAK	110	3.1	20.4	1.8	2.6
Tikka PATAK	141	3.6	16.9	6.5	3.5
Curry Sauce canned	78	1.5	7.1	5	n/a
jar HELLMANN'S	87	0.8	21.1	Tr	1.6
Medium UNCLE BEN'S	66	0.9	10.9	2	n/a
Delhi Tomato & Coriander Cooking Sauce PATAK	158	2	8.9	12.7	1.9
Dhansak Cooking Sauce					
LOYD GROSSMAN	82	3.4	11.1	2.7	n/a
SHARWOOD	100	4.5	13.8	3	3.5

All amounts per 100g/100ml unless otherwise stated	Cal kcal	Pro g	Carb g	Fat g	Fibre g
Dopiaza Cooking Sauce					
LOYD GROSSMAN	**92**	2.4	12.9	3.4	n/a
PATAK	**112**	1.6	9.8	7.3	1.2
SHARWOOD	**85**	1.4	10.1	4.3	2.2
Goan Pineapple Cooking Sauce					
PATAK	**128**	1.5	6.4	10.6	0.3
Kashmiri Cooking Sauce					
SHARWOOD	**110**	3	13	5.1	1.5
Masala Cooking Sauce					
WEIGHT WATCHERS	**55**	1.4	8.6	1.7	0.8
Jalfrezi Cooking Sauce					
LOYD GROSSMAN	**127**	2.1	8.2	9.5	n/a
PATAK	**116**	1.7	11.3	7	1.4
SHARWOOD	**76**	1.1	8.1	4.2	1.2
grilled pepper PATAK	**99**	1.3	7.8	7	1.2
Karai Cooking Sauce PATAK	**126**	4	15.7	5.2	1.1
Korma Sizzle & Stir KNORR	**246**	1.5	10.3	22.1	1.3
Korma Cooking Sauce					
LOYD GROSSMAN	**244**	3.6	19.1	17	n/a
SHARWOOD	**136**	1.6	14.7	7.8	2.2
UNCLE BEN'S	**126**	1.4	11.1	8.4	n/a
orange zest PATAK	**171**	1.8	8.5	14.4	0.9
organic MERIDIAN FOODS LTD	**136**	2.4	9	9.9	1.7
reduced fat, sugar & salt SHARWOOD	**103**	1.5	10	6.3	3

All amounts per 100g/100ml unless otherwise stated	Cal kcal	Pro g	Carb g	Fat g	Fibre g
Waistline CROSSE & BLACKWELL with coconut flakes & fresh	**104**	1.9	14.7	4.2	n/a
cream, Just for One UNCLE BEN'S	**132**	1.5	11	9	n/a
Korma Cook-in-Sauce HOMEPRIDE	**154**	1.9	11.9	11	1.3
Madras Cooking Sauce					
LOYD GROSSMAN	**180**	2.5	6.8	15.9	n/a
SHARWOOD	**100**	1.9	7.9	6.7	3.9
reduced fat, sugar & salt					
SHARWOOD	**68**	1.7	5.7	4.3	4.3
Makhani Cooking Sauce					
SHARWOOD	**111**	1.2	10	7.4	1.9
Pasanda Cooking Sauce PATAK	**157**	2.3	9.2	12.2	0.5
SHARWOOD	**159**	3.3	12.4	10.7	1.6
Rogan Josh Cooking Sauce					
LOYD GROSSMAN	**194**	2.4	10.5	15.8	n/a
SHARWOOD	**71**	1.5	7.7	3.8	3.5
organic PATAK	**96**	1	7.3	7	0.6
red wine PATAK	**104**	1.1	7.2	6.8	0.9
with tomato UNCLE BEN'S	**61**	1.3	7.7	2.7	0.5
Tandoori Cooking Sauce					
SHARWOOD	**133**	2.9	18.1	5.4	2.1
Tikka Bhuna Sizzle & Stir KNORR	**116**	1.2	6.7	9.4	1.1
Tikka Masala Cooking Sauce					
LOYD GROSSMAN	**206**	2.6	12.5	16.2	n/a

All amounts per 100g/100ml unless otherwise stated	Cal kcal	Pro g	Carb g	Fat g	Fibre g
SHARWOOD	**116**	1.7	9.8	7.7	1.6
UNCLE BEN'S	**98**	1.4	8.8	6.4	n/a
low carbohydrate CARB OPTIONS	**73**	1.5	4	5.7	1.3
organic MERIDIAN FOODS LTD	**129**	1.8	10.7	8.7	1.1
reduced fat, sugar & salt SHARWOOD	**79**	1.5	6.9	5	2.5
saffron PATAK	**105**	1.3	7.9	7.5	1
spicy SHARWOOD	**116**	1.6	11.3	7.1	2.4
Waistline CROSSE & BLACKWELL	**82**	2.9	11.2	2.8	n/a
Tikka Masala Cook-in-Sauce					
HOMEPRIDE	**146**	1.7	10.6	10.7	1.4
Tikka Masala Sizzle & Stir KNORR	**190**	1.5	8.8	16.6	1.4
Tikka Stir it Up KNORR	**654**	6.3	18.6	61.6	2.1
Vindaloo PATAK	**119**	1.7	8.5	8.6	2.1

MEXICAN & US

Barbecue Cook-In-Sauce					
HOMEPRIDE	**83**	0.8	16.2	1.7	0.5
Barbecue Sauce, Texas Hot					
KNORR	**306**	6.2	66.4	1.3	3.4
Buffalo Wings Sauce					
DISCOVERY FOODS	**62**	n/a	8.8	2.4	n/a
Cajun Sauce UNCLE BEN'S	**56**	1	8.2	2	n/a

All amounts per 100g/100ml unless otherwise stated	Cal kcal	Pro g	Carb g	Fat g	Fibre g
Cajun Seasoning Mix					
DISCOVERY FOODS	190	n/a	36	4.5	n/a
Californian Lemon Pepper					
Stir it Up KNORR	659	5.2	26.1	59.3	2.7
Chicken Fahitas Mexican Creations					
Mix, as sold					
CROSSE & BLACKWELL	310	11.4	48.4	7.1	3.5
Chicken Fajita Dry Casserole Mix,					
as sold COLMAN'S	344	9.4	62.5	6.3	4.8
SCHWARTZ	325	10.4	63.3	3.3	0.5
Chilli Con Carne Sizzle & Stir					
KNORR	117	2.6	9.9	7.5	1.7
Chilli con Carne Dry Casserole Mix,					
as sold COLMAN'S	318	7.9	67.4	1.9	4.9
hot, as sold COLMAN'S	314	9.4	63.7	2.4	6
medium SCHWARTZ	308	8.2	64.6	1.9	0.5
Chilli con Carne Mexican Creations					
Mix, as sold CROSSE & BLACKWELL	320	14	32.3	14.6	8.8
Chilli Cook-In-Sauce HOMEPRIDE	53	1.5	10.3	0.6	1.4
Chilli Sauce					
Hot UNCLE BEN'S	51	2	9.6	0.4	n/a
Medium UNCLE BEN'S	58	1.8	10.8	0.8	n/a
Creole Sauce DISCOVERY FOODS	88	n/a	16.6	19	n/a

All amounts per 100g/100ml unless otherwise stated	Cal kcal	Pro g	Carb g	Fat g	Fibre g
Enchilada Cooking Sauce					
OLD EL PASO	**81.7**	1.2	10.4	4	n/a
Enchilada Sauce DISCOVERY FOODS	**35**	n/a	2.5	2.5	n/a
Fajita Cooking Sauce, Smoky BBQ flavour OLD EL PASO	**39.8**	1.6	8.4	0.5	n/a
Fajita Seasoning Mix					
DISCOVERY FOODS	**270**	n/a	53	7	n/a
OLD EL PASO	**306**	9	54	6	n/a
Mexican Chili Chicken Mix					
SCHWARTZ	**327**	7.9	63.6	4.5	5.8
Mexican Chilli Cooking Sauce					
WEIGHT WATCHERS	**37**	1.5	7	0.3	1.2
Mexican Fajita Stir it Up KNORR	**651**	5.3	19.7	61.2	3.6
Mexican Sauce DISCOVERY FOODS	**89**	n/a	12.3	3.8	n/a
Ranch Barbecue Sausages Tonight Sauce KNORR	**75**	1.5	17.2	0.1	0.9
Sticky Ribs Sauce DISCOVERY FOODS	**164**	n/a	37.3	1.1	n/a
Taco Seasoning Mix					
DISCOVERY FOODS	**316**	n/a	61.5	5.5	n/a
OLD EL PASO	**336**	6	69	4	n/a
Texan Barbeque Stir it Up KNORR	**626**	4.2	29.5	54.6	1.6
Texas BBQ with Sweet Peppers Sauce UNCLE BEN'S	**75**	1.1	16	0.6	n/a

All amounts per 100g/100ml unless otherwise stated	Cal kcal	Pro g	Carb g	Fat g	Fibre g
EUROPEAN					
Beef Bourguignon Dry					
Casserole Mix, as sold COLMAN'S	**308**	4.9	68.6	1.6	2.2
Beef Stroganoff Dry Casserole					
Mix, as sold COLMAN'S	**350**	11.6	56.1	8.9	2.7
Chasseur Cook-In-Sauce					
HOMEPRIDE	**41**	0.7	9.2	0.1	0.4
Chicken Chasseur Dry Casserole					
Mix, as sold COLMAN'S	**284**	8	59.2	1.6	3.8
Classic Chasseur Chicken					
Tonight Sauce KNORR	**48**	0.5	4.6	3.1	0.6
Coq au Vin Dry Casserole Mix,					
as sold COLMAN'S	**301**	5.5	65.6	1.8	3.3
Country French Chicken					
Tonight Sauce KNORR	**90**	0.5	4.1	8	0.7
low fat	**45**	0.4	4.4	2.9	0.7
Dijonnaise Pan Fry Sauce					
LOYD GROSSMAN	**81**	2.1	4.9	5.9	n/a
Roasted Garlic & Thyme Pourover					
Dry Sauce Mix, as sold KNORR	**314**	6.8	63.5	3.7	3.7
Spanish Chicken Chicken					
Tonight Sauce KNORR	**46**	1.5	7	1.4	0.6

All amounts per 100g/100ml unless otherwise stated	Cal kcal	Pro g	Carb g	Fat g	Fibre g
Spanish Chicken with Sun-Ripened Tomato Sauce UNCLE BEN'S	39	1	7	0.7	0.6
Spicy Sauce CARB OPTIONS	27	1.4	5	0.1	0.9

WORLD

Indonesian Satay Sauce SHARWOOD	159	5.4	10	10.8	5.1
Jamaican Jerk Stir it Up KNORR	633	3.9	20.9	59.3	5.4
Mild Thai Curry with Lime & Coconut, as sold GO ORGANIC	125	1.6	6.2	10.4	1.2
Moroccan Tagine Pan Fry Sauce LOYD GROSSMAN	58	1.1	5.9	3.3	n/a
Moroccan Tajine with Saffron Sauce UNCLE BEN'S	60	0.9	12.2	0.9	0.4
Satay Sauce					
Just for One UNCLE BEN'S	160	4.5	13.8	9.2	0.5
Oriental Sauces LOYD GROSSMAN	231	5.7	14.7	16.6	n/a
Stir Fry AMOY	294	7.9	25.5	17.8	n/a
Singapore Laksa Sauce SHARWOOD	131	1.4	7.2	13.2	2.9
Teriyaki with Black Pepper Stir-Fry Sauce SHARWOOD	96	0.9	22.5	0.3	0.3
Thai Chilli Sauce SHARWOOD	164	1.8	39.1	Tr	0.3

All amounts per 100g/100ml unless otherwise stated	Cal kcal	Pro g	Carb g	Fat g	Fibre g
Thai Coriander Marinade					
LEA & PERRINS	**147**	0.8	29.5	3	0.5
Thai Coconut Curry Sauce					
UNCLE BEN'S	**101**	1.4	13.2	4.8	n/a
Thai Green Curry Sauce					
LOYD GROSSMAN	**104**	1.6	10	6.4	n/a
SHARWOOD	**123**	1.2	4	11.3	2
Sizzle & Stir KNORR	**212**	0.8	6.6	20.3	0.7
with coconut & lemongrass, Just for One UNCLE BEN'S	**77**	1.2	5.8	5.5	n/a
with coriander & lime GO ORGANIC	**124**	1.6	6.3	10.3	1.3
Thai Red Curry Sauce					
LOYD GROSSMAN	**125**	2.8	13.7	6.5	n/a
SHARWOOD	**131**	1.4	5.8	11.3	2
with galangal & red chili GO ORGANIC	**99**	1.6	5.5	7.8	1.3
Thai Sweet Chilli Sauce					
LOYD GROSSMAN	**140**	1.8	32.7	0.2	n/a
UNCLE BEN'S	**98**	0.9	23	0.3	n/a
Thai Yellow Sauce LOYD GROSSMAN	**111**	1.7	9.1	7.5	n/a

CRISPS & NIBBLES

All amounts per 100g/100ml unless otherwise stated	Cal kcal	Pro g	Carb g	Fat g	Fibre g
CRISPS					
Barbecue Flavour Crisps,					
per pack (34.5g) WALKERS	**181**	2.2	17.3	11.4	1.4
Beef & Onion Crisps,					
per pack (34.5g) WALKERS	**181**	2.2	17.3	11.4	1.4
Big Cheese Wheat Crunchies,					
per pack (35g) GOLDEN WONDER	**172**	3.3	19.8	8.8	1.1
Cheese & Onion Crisps, per pack					
(34.5g) GOLDEN WONDER	**176**	2.1	17.9	10.7	1.6
(34.5g) WALKERS	**181**	2.2	17.3	11.4	1.4
Lites (28g) WALKERS	**130**	2.1	17.1	5.9	1.4
Crispy Bacon Wheat Crunchies,					
per pack (35g) GOLDEN WONDER	**172**	3.4	19.6	8.9	1.4
Grilled Chicken Golden Lights,					
per pack (21g) GOLDEN WONDER	**93**	0.9	13.9	3.8	0.9
Honey Glazed Ham Flavour Crisps,					
Lites (28g) WALKERS	**112**	1.7	14.9	0.5	1.2
Hula Hoops, per pack (27g)					
all flavours UNITED BISCUITS	**175**	1.1	20.5	9.7	0.6
Loaded Cheese Golden Skins,					
per pack (45g) GOLDEN WONDER	**232**	2.7	22.9	14.3	n/a
Kettle Chips KETTLE FOODS					
Feta Cheese & Olive,					
Mediterranean	**495**	7.3	50.3	29.4	5.3

All amounts per 100g/100ml unless otherwise stated	Cal kcal	Pro g	Carb g	Fat g	Fibre g
Lightly Salted	**485**	6.3	55.1	26.6	5.2
Mango Chilli	**475**	6.3	53.9	24	6.1
Mature Cheddar & Chive	**478**	8.1	54.4	25.4	5
Salsa with Mesquite	**462**	5.8	55.2	24.2	5.7
Sea Salt & Balsamic Vinegar	**489**	6.8	53.5	27.5	4.9
Sea Salt with Crushed Black Peppercorns	**482**	6.5	53.8	26.7	4.9
Sweet Chilli	**468**	7.3	51.4	25.9	6.3
Sweet Red Pepper & Sun Dried Tomato	**490**	6.3	53.3	27.9	5
Yoghurt & Green Onion	**486**	6.1	54.7	27	4.3
Undressed	**486**	56.3	5.9	26.3	5
Mediterranean Tomato & Basil Golden Lights, per pack (150g) GOLDEN WONDER	**111**	1	16.5	4.5	1.1
Mexican Chilli & Cheese Golden Skins, per pack (45g) GOLDEN WONDER	**231**	3	22.8	14.1	n/a
Pepperoni & Cheese Golden Skins, per pack (45g) GOLDEN WONDER	**231**	2.8	22.9	14.2	n/a
Pickled Onion Crisps, per pack (34.5g) GOLDEN WONDER	**173**	1.9	17.6	10.6	1.6
Potato Crisps	**530**	5.7	53.3	34.2	n/a
low fat	**458**	6.6	63.5	21.5	n/a

All amounts per 100g/100ml unless otherwise stated	Cal kcal	Pro g	Carb g	Fat g	Fibre g
Quavers, per pack (20g) WALKERS					
cheese	**103**	0.6	12.2	5.8	0.2
prawn cocktail	**84**	0.4	10	4.6	0.2
salt & vinegar	**82**	0.4	9.5	4.8	0.2
Ready Salted Crisps, per pack					
(34.5g) GOLDEN WONDER	**179**	1.9	17.8	11.1	1.6
(34.5g) WALKERS	**183**	2.2	16.9	11.7	1.4
Lites (28g) WALKERS	**132**	2.1	16.8	6.2	1.4
Ringos, per pack (34g) GOLDEN WONDER					
cheese & onion	**81**	1.2	11.6	3.3	0.6
pickled onion	**79**	1	11.3	3.3	0.5
salt & vinegar	**79**	1	11.4	3.3	0.5
Roast Chicken Crisps, per pack					
(34.5g) GOLDEN WONDER	**176**	2.1	17.9	10.7	1.7
Salt & Black Pepper Golden Skins,					
per pack (45g) GOLDEN WONDER	**232**	2.7	23.6	14	n/a
Salt & Vinegar Crisps, per pack					
(34.5g) GOLDEN WONDER	**173**	1.8	17.7	10.6	1.5
(34.5g) WALKERS	**181**	2.2	17.3	11.4	1.4
Golden Lights (21g)					
GOLDEN WONDER	**93**	0.8	13.8	3.8	0.9
Lites (28g) WALKERS	**112**	1.8	14.6	5	1.2
Salt & Vinegar Golden Skins,					
per pack (45g) GOLDEN WONDER	**228**	2.6	22.8	14	n/a

All amounts per 100g/100ml unless otherwise stated	Cal kcal	Pro g	Carb g	Fat g	Fibre g
Sausage & Tomato Crisps, per pack					
(34.5g) GOLDEN WONDER	**175**	2.1	17.7	10.6	1.5
Sea Salt Golden Lights,					
per pack (21g) GOLDEN WONDER	**94**	0.8	13.9	3.9	0.9
Sour Cream & Onion Golden Lights,					
per pack (21g) GOLDEN WONDER	**93**	0.9	13.9	3.8	0.9
Spicy Tomato Wheat Crunchies,					
per pack (35g) GOLDEN WONDER	**172**	3.3	19.6	8.9	1.4
Tomato Ketchup Crisps, per pack					
(34.5g) GOLDEN WONDER	**175**	1.8	18.3	10.5	1.6
Worcester Sauce Wheat Crunchies,					
per pack (35g) GOLDEN WONDER	**172**	3.3	19.7	8.9	1.4
Wotsits, per pack (21g) WALKERS					
Cheesy	**110**	1.7	11.3	6.3	0.2
Flamin' Hot	**109**	1.1	12	6.3	0.3
Mild Cheese (19g)	**102**	1.1	10.3	6.3	0.2
Prawn Cocktail (19g)	**99**	1	10.5	5.9	0.2
Twisted BBQ (22g)	**113**	1	12.5	6.6	0.3
Twisted Really Cheesy (22g)	**117**	1.3	12.1	7	0.2

See also: **KIDS' FOODS**

NIBBLES

Bites, Italian JACOB'S	**504**	8.4	53.4	28.5	4.2
Bites, rib 'n saucy JACOB'S	**511**	8.2	56	28.2	2.3

All amounts per 100g/100ml unless otherwise stated	Cal kcal	Pro g	Carb g	Fat g	Fibre g
Bombay Mix HOLLAND & BARRETT	**507**	11.2	38.3	34.3	10.6
Cashews					
salted	**615**	20	19	51	3.2
kernel only, roasted, salted					
HOLLAND & BARRETT	**611**	20.5	18.8	50.9	3.2
whole nuts HOLLAND & BARRETT	**573**	17.7	18.2	48.2	9.5
Doritos, per pack (40g) WALKERS					
cool original	**202**	3	23.2	10.8	1.2
extreme chilli heatwave	**196**	2.6	23.2	10.4	1.2
tangy cheese	**202**	3.4	22.8	10.8	1.4
Doritos Dippas, Dipping Chip, lightly salted WALKERS	**490**	7.5	63	23	3.5
hint of chilli	**495**	7	61	25	3.5
hint of lime	**495**	7	61	25	3.5
Japanese Rice Crackers					
HOLLAND & BARRETT	**400**	9.4	78.9	5.2	0.5
Lite Bites KELLOGG'S					
Cheese	**416**	9	77	8	1
Tikka	**416**	7	79	8	1.5
Tomato	**416**	7	79	8	1.5
Macadamia Nuts, salted	**748**	7.9	4.8	77.6	n/a
Nachos Kit OLD EL PASO					
Nachips	**506**	7	61	26	n/a
topping	**64**	3	13	0	n/a

All amounts per 100g/100ml unless otherwise stated	Cal kcal	Pro g	Carb g	Fat g	Fibre g
Nik Naks, per pack (34g) GOLDEN WONDER					
cream 'n' cheesy	196	1.8	17.9	13	0.1
nice 'n' spicy	193	1.5	17.9	12.8	0.1
rib 'n' saucy	194	1.5	18.3	12.8	0.2
scampi 'n' lemon	194	1.7	18.1	12.8	Tr
Peanuts, dry roasted	590	25.7	10.3	49.8	n/a
roasted & salted	602	24.7	7.1	53	n/a
Peanuts & Raisins	436	15.4	37.5	25.9	N
blanched HOLLAND & BARRETT	473	17.6	31.8	30.6	4.8
yogurt coated HOLLAND & BARRETT	465	8.9	54.3	25.8	2
Pistachio Nuts, roasted & salted	599	18	8	55	6
Popcorn candied	480	2.1	77.6	20	n/a
plain	593	6.2	48.7	42.8	n/a
uncooked HOLLAND & BARRETT	592	6.2	48.6	42.8	Tr
Poppadums					
fried in veg. oil	369	17.5	39.1	16.9	N
cracked black pepper SHARWOOD	461	16.7	32.7	27.3	7.3
garlic & coriander SHARWOOD	438	18.4	43	21.4	6.5
garlic & green chilli SHARWOOD	268	23.2	39.4	1.9	14.6
plain PATAK	417	16.7	60	12.2	n/a
plain SHARWOOD	273	21.9	45.7	0.3	10.1
spicy SHARWOOD	257	20.2	43	0.5	13
Prawn Crackers SHARWOOD	309	0.7	41.2	15.7	1.2
Scooples KAVLI					
original	380	13.9	77.9	1.4	3

All amounts per 100g/100ml unless otherwise stated	Cal kcal	Pro g	Carb g	Fat g	Fibre g
garlic	**341**	11.5	76.8	1.9	7.4
tomato	**352**	11.5	75.6	2.5	4.5
wholemeal	**386**	11.9	83.2	0.6	7.7
Snack-a-Jacks QUAKER					
caramel flavour	**401**	5.5	86	3.5	0.5
cheese flavour	**383**	8	81	3	1
chocolate chip	**408**	5.5	81	6.5	1.5
chocolate orange	**394**	5.5	83	4.5	1
Snack-a-Jacks, per pack (30g) QUAKER					
barbecue	**125**	2.1	24	2.1	0.3
cheese	**123**	2.4	22.5	2.6	0.3
prawn cocktail	**122**	2	22.9	2.4	0.3
roast chicken	**123**	2.1	23.2	2.4	0.3
salt & vinegar	**123**	2	23	2.4	0.3
smoked ham	**114**	1.8	21.9	2.1	0.6
sour cream & chive	**123**	2.3	23.1	2.4	0.3
Snack-a-Jacks Mini Bites per pack (28g) QUAKER					
mature cheddar & red onion	**116**	2.1	21.3	2.5	0.6
smoked ham	**114**	1.8	21.9	2.1	0.6
sour cream & sweet chilli	**114**	1.8	21.7	2.2	0.6
Thai Bites JACOB'S					
oriental spice	**397**	7.3	82.5	4.2	0.2
seaweed	**377**	7.1	80	3.2	0.5
Tortilla Chips	**459**	7.6	60.1	22.6	n/a
Chili flavour OLD EL PASO	**496**	7	62	26	n/a

All amounts per 100g/100ml unless otherwise stated	Cal kcal	Pro g	Carb g	Fat g	Fibre g
gluten-free DISCOVERY FOODS	485	n/a	65.3	21.8	n/a
Jalapeño Cheese flavour OLD EL PASO	520	7	61	27	n/a
Lousiana Hot Sauce flavour KETTLE FOODS	485	7.5	59.2	24.2	4.9
Mexicana Cheddar flavour KETTLE FOODS	501	7.7	57.4	26.7	3.3
Salsa flavour OLD EL PASO	494	7	65	26	n/a
Spicy Enchilada flavour KETTLE FOODS	497	7.3	54	28	4
Trail Mix	432	9.1	37.2	28.5	n/a
Twiglets JACOB'S	384	12.3	57.3	11.7	11.3

DAIRY PRODUCTS

All amounts per 100g/100ml unless otherwise stated	Cal kcal	Pro g	Carb g	Fat g	Fibre g
MILK & CREAM					
Buttermilk, cultured St Ivel	**55**	5.7	8.1	Tr	n/a
Cream					
extra thick Nestlé	**233**	2.6	3.6	23.1	0
extra thick, organic Yeo Valley	**294**	2.3	3.6	30	0
fresh, clotted	**586**	1.6	2.3	63.5	n/a
fresh, double	**496**	1.6	1.7	53.7	0
fresh, double, organic Yeo Valley	**459**	1.7	2.8	49	0
fresh, half	**162**	2.7	4.4	15	0
fresh, single	**193**	3.3	2.2	19.1	0
fresh, soured	**205**	2.9	3.8	19.9	n/a
fresh, whipping	**381**	2	2.7	40.3	0
sterilised, canned	**239**	2.5	3.7	23.9	n/a
UHT, aerosol spray	**252**	1.9	7.2	24.2	0
UHT, double Elmlea	**305**	2.5	4	31	0.5
UHT, double, light Elmlea	**231**	2.5	3.5	23	0.3
UHT, single Elmlea	**148**	3.1	4.6	13	0.2
UHT, single, light Elmlea	**117**	3.1	4.8	9.5	0.5
UHT, Squirty (aerosol) Elmlea	**254**	1.5	6.3	24.8	Tr
UHT, whipping Elmlea	**285**	2.4	3.5	29	0.2
Crème fraiche					
full fat	**378**	2.2	2.4	40	0
half fat	**162**	2.7	4.4	15	0
organic Yeo Valley	**178**	2.1	3.1	17.5	0
Milk, fresh					
cows', whole, average	**66**	3.3	4.5	3.9	n/a

All amounts per 100g/100ml unless otherwise stated	Cal kcal	Pro g	Carb g	Fat g	Fibre g
cows', whole, organic YEO VALLEY	68	3.4	4.7	4	0
cows', semi-skimmed, average	46	3.4	4.7	1.7	0
cows', semi-skimmed, organic YEO VALLEY	47	3.6	4.8	1.8	0
cows', skimmed, average	32	3.4	4.4	0.2	0
cows', Channel Island	78	3.6	4.8	5.1	n/a
goats', pasteurised	62	3.1	4.4	3.7	0
sheep's, raw	93	5.4	5.1	5.8	0
Milk, evaporated NESTLÉ					
Carnation	160	8.2	11.5	9	0
Carnation Light	110	7.5	10.5	4	0
Milk, dried					
skimmed	348	36.1	52.9	0.6	0
skimmed, as sold MARVEL	361	36.1	52.9	0.6	n/a
made up with water MARVEL	206	20.6	30.2	0.3	n/a
Milk, condensed					
wholemilk, sweetened	333	8.5	55.5	10.1	n/a
skimmed milk, sweetened	267	10	60	0.2	n/a
tin NESTLÉ	330	8.3	54.3	9.1	0
tin, light NESTLÉ	267	10	60	0.2	0
Pro.active Milk Drink FLORA	49	3.6	4.7	1.8	0
Soya Milk					
chocolate, organic PROVAMEL	81	3.8	10.7	2.4	1.2
sweetened	43	3.1	2.5	2.4	Tr
sweetened, organic PROVAMEL	46	3.7	2.8	2.2	0.6

All amounts per 100g/100ml unless otherwise stated	Cal kcal	Pro g	Carb g	Fat g	Fibre g
unsweetened	26	2.4	0.5	1.6	0.5
unsweetened, organic PROVAMEL	35	3.7	0.1	2.2	0.6
Rice Drink PROVAMEL					
calcium enriched	50	0.1	9.6	1.2	0
organic	49	0.1	9.5	1.2	0

YOGURT & FROMAGE FRAIS

Non-branded Yogurt

	Cal kcal	Pro g	Carb g	Fat g	Fibre g
Greek-style, cows, fruit	137	4.8	11.2	8.4	Tr
Greek-style, cows, plain	133	5.7	4.8	10.2	0
Greek-style, sheep	92	4.8	5	6	0
low fat, fruit	78	4.2	13.7	1.1	0.3
low fat, plain	56	4.8	7.4	1	N
soya, fruit	73	2.1	12.9	1.8	0.7
virtually fat free, fruit	47	4.8	7	0.2	Tr
virtually fat free, plain	54	5.4	8.2	0.2	0
whole milk, fruit	109	4	17.7	3	N
whole milk, plain	79	5.7	7.8	3	N

Non-branded Fromage Frais

	Cal kcal	Pro g	Carb g	Fat g	Fibre g
fruit	124	5.3	13.9	5.6	Tr
plain	113	6.1	4.4	8	0
vitually fat free, fruit	50	6.8	5.6	0.2	0.7
vitually fat free, plain	49	7.7	4.6	0.1	0

Amoré Luxury Yogurts MÜLLER

	Cal kcal	Pro g	Carb g	Fat g	Fibre g
Apple Strudel	141	2.4	15.4	7.8	n/a

All amounts per 100g/100ml unless otherwise stated	Cal kcal	Pro g	Carb g	Fat g	Fibre g
Creamy Cappuccino with Stracciatelli	**159**	2.4	16.2	9.4	n/a
Morello Cherry	**137**	2.2	15.5	7.4	n/a
Spanish Orange	**145**	2.3	16.3	7.8	n/a
Walnut & Greek Honey	**151**	2.3	16.1	8.6	n/a
Apple & Banana Bio Yogurt HOLLAND & BARRETT	**54**	4.4	5.6	1.5	0
Apricot & Mango TropicYogurt SKI	**95**	4.5	15.4	1.7	0.1
Apricot & Passion Fruit Fat Free Yogurt, organic YEO VALLEY	**76**	5.2	13.6	0.1	0.1
Apricot Flavour Pro.active Yoghurt FLORA	**78**	3.9	14.5	0.5	0.2
Apricot Tart Yogurt SVELTESSE	**78**	4.8	14.2	0.2	0.1
Apricot Yogurt Wholemilk, organic YEO VALLEY	**101**	4.1	12.4	3.9	0.1
Blackberry Yogurt SVELTESSE	**55**	4.7	8.8	0.1	0.3
Black Cherry Yogurt SKI	**99**	4.5	16.3	1.7	0.1
Blackcurrant Wholemilk Yogurt, organic YEO VALLEY	**101**	4.1	12.4	3.9	0.2
Caramelised Apple Yogurt SVELTESSE	**59**	4.7	9.3	0.3	0.2
Cherry Flavour Pro.active Yoghurt FLORA	**81**	3.9	15.2	0.5	0.1

All amounts per 100g/100ml unless otherwise stated	Cal kcal	Pro g	Carb g	Fat g	Fibre g
Cherry Yogurt SHAPE	**47**	4.6	6.8	0.1	2.1
Citrus Fruit Yogurts, fat free					
WEIGHT WATCHERS	**41**	4	5.8	0.1	Tr
Fruit Corner MÜLLER					
blackberry & raspberry	**110**	3.7	15	3.9	n/a
blueberry	**112**	3.7	15.5	3.9	n/a
cherry	**110**	3.7	15	3.9	n/a
peach & apricot	**110**	3.7	15	3.9	n/a
raspberry	**114**	4.2	15.3	4	n/a
strawberry	**118**	3.7	17.1	3.9	n/a
Goats' Milk Yogurt					
HOLLAND & BARRETT	**60**	3.3	4.4	3.5	Tr
Greek Style Yogurt YEO VALLEY					
Natural, organic	**136**	4.7	6.9	10	0
Honey, organic	**153**	4	15.2	8.5	0
Strawberry, organic	**146**	4.1	13.3	8.5	0.2
Guava & Orange Fat Free					
Yogurt, organic YEO VALLEY	**74**	5.1	13.2	0.1	0.3
Lemon Cheesecake Yogurt					
SVELTESSE	**81**	4.6	13.8	0.7	0.1
Mango Yogurt SHAPE	**46**	4.6	6.7	0.1	2.1
Müllerlight MÜLLER					
apple pie flavoured yogurt	**64**	4.6	10.9	0.2	n/a
blackcurrant yogurt	**55**	4.7	8.9	0.1	n/a

All amounts per 100g/100ml unless otherwise stated	Cal kcal	Pro g	Carb g	Fat g	Fibre g
cherry yogurt	**50**	4.4	7.9	0.1	n/a
chocolate yogurt	**66**	4.7	11	0.3	n/a
country berries yogurt	**52**	4.4	8.3	0.1	n/a
lemon cheesecake flavoured yogurt	**64**	4.7	10.9	0.2	n/a
mandarin yogurt	**54**	4.3	9	0.1	n/a
peach & maracuya yogurt	**50**	4.4	7.9	0.1	n/a
pineapple & peach yogurt	**53**	4.4	8.7	0.1	n/a
raspberry & cranberry yogurt	**53**	4.4	8.7	0.1	n/a
rhubarb crumble flavoured yogurt	**64**	4.7	10.9	0.2	n/a
strawberry cheesecake flavoured yogurt	**65**	4.7	11.1	0.2	n/a
strawberry yogurt	**53**	4.4	8.7	0.1	n/a
toffee yogurt	**53**	4.4	8.5	0.1	n/a
vanilla yogurt	**53**	4.6	8.3	0.1	n/a
Natural Bio Yogurt					
HOLLAND & BARRETT	**54**	4.4	5.6	1.5	0
Natural Yogurt					
creamy, thick WEIGHT WATCHERS	**142**	4.9	5.3	0.1	Tr
fat free, organic YEO VALLEY	**58**	5.9	8.4	0.1	n/a
organic YEO VALLEY	**82**	4.5	6.6	4.2	0
Nectarine & Passionfruit Yogurt					
SHAPE	**46**	4.6	6.7	0.1	2.1
Orange & Guava Tropic Yogurt					
SKI	**95**	4.5	15.5	1.7	0.2

All amounts per 100g/100ml unless otherwise stated	Cal kcal	Pro g	Carb g	Fat g	Fibre g
Peach & Apricot Yogurt SHAPE	**46**	4.6	6.7	0.1	2.1
Peach & Papaya Fat Free Yogurt, organic YEO VALLEY	**76**	5.1	13.6	0.1	0.1
Peach & Passionfruit Tropic Yogurt SKI	**95**	4.6	15.4	1.7	0.1
Peach Fat Free Yogurt SKI	**79**	4.5	15.1	0.1	0.2
Peach Melba Yogurt SVELTESSE	**56**	4.7	9.1	0.1	0.2
Pineapple & Mango Fat Free Yogurt, organic YEO VALLEY	**77**	5.1	13.9	0.1	0.1
Pineapple & Papaya Tropic Yogurt SKI	**95**	4.5	15.4	1.7	0.1
Plum Fat Free Yogurt, organic YEO VALLEY	**78**	5.1	14.2	0.1	0.1
Plum Wholemilk Yogurt, organic YEO VALLEY	**101**	4.1	12.4	3.9	0.1
Raspberry Flavour Pro.active Yoghurt FLORA	**78**	3.9	14.4	0.5	0.5
Raspberry Wholemilk Yogurt, organic YEO VALLEY	**101**	4.2	12.3	3.9	0.4
Raspberry Yogurt fat free SKI	**81**	4.7	15.4	0.1	0.5
fat free, organic YEO VALLEY	**78**	5.2	14	0.1	0.4
smooth SHAPE	**46**	4.6	6.7	0.1	2.2
SKI	**96**	4.9	15.1	1.8	0.1

All amounts per 100g/100ml unless otherwise stated	Cal kcal	Pro g	Carb g	Fat g	Fibre g
Red Fruits Crumble Yogurt					
SVELTESSE	**55**	4.3	9	0.2	0.2
Rhubarb Crumble Yogurt					
SVELTESSE	**77**	4.8	14.1	0.2	0.3
Rhubarb Yogurt SKI	**92**	4.5	14.6	1.7	0.2
Red Cherry Fat Free Yogurt SKI	**79**	4.5	15.1	0.1	0.2
Strawberry Bio Yogurt					
HOLLAND & BARRETT	**54**	4.4	5.6	1.5	0
Solo Pots SHAPE					
Blissful Blackberry	**43**	4.6	5.9	0.1	2.1
Really Raspberry	**43**	4.6	5.9	0.1	2.2
Sumptuous Strawberry	**43**	4.5	5.9	0.1	2.1
Strawberry Yogurt SHAPE	**46**	4.6	6.7	0.1	2.1
SVELTESSE	**56**	4.7	9.1	0.1	0.2
fat free SKI	**80**	4.5	15.2	0.1	0.2
low fat, organic YEO VALLEY	**77**	5.1	14	0.1	0.1
smooth SKI	**96**	4.8	15.1	1.8	0.1
Strawberry Smoothies YEO VALLEY					
Strawberry, organic	**100**	4.1	12.2	3.9	0.1
Strawberry & Blackberry, organic	**100**	4.1	12.2	3.9	0.1
Strawberry & Raspberry, organic	**100**	4.1	12.2	3.9	0.2
Strawberry & Vanilla, organic	**100**	4.1	12.3	3.9	0.1
Strawberry Wholemilk Yogurt, organic YEO VALLEY	**101**	4.1	12.3	3.9	0.1

All amounts per 100g/100ml unless otherwise stated	Cal kcal	Pro g	Carb g	Fat g	Fibre g
Summer Fruits Yogurts, low fat					
WEIGHT WATCHERS					
Black Cherry	**48**	4.2	7.5	0.1	0.1
Peach	**46**	4.2	7.1	0.1	0.2
Raspberry	**49**	5.1	6.8	0.1	0.3
Strawberry	**43**	4.1	6.2	0.1	0.1
Toffee Flavour Yogurts, fat free					
WEIGHT WATCHERS	**40**	3.9	5.9	0.1	0.8
Toffee Fat Free Yogurt,					
organic YEO VALLEY	**92**	5.1	17.6	0.1	0
Toffee Fromage Frais					
WEIGHT WATCHERS	**59**	5.2	9.3	0.1	1
Tropical Fruits Yogurts, low fat					
WEIGHT WATCHERS					
Mango	**45**	3.9	7.1	0.1	1.1
Melon & Passionfruit	**45**	4	7	0.1	Tr
Pineapple & Coconut	**47**	3.9	7.4	0.1	0.1
Pineapple	**47**	3.9	7.7	0.1	0.9
Vanilla Fat Free Yogurt,					
organic YEO VALLEY	**84**	5.3	15.4	0.1	0
Vanilla Flavour Yogurts,					
fat free WEIGHT WATCHERS	**42**	3.9	6.5	0.1	Tr
Vanilla Fromage Frais					
WEIGHT WATCHERS	**49**	5.3	6.9	0.1	1.2

All amounts per 100g/100ml unless otherwise stated	Cal kcal	Pro g	Carb g	Fat g	Fibre g
Very Berry Yogurt SKI					
fruits of the forest	**95**	4.5	15.5	1.7	0.4
raspberry & cranberry	**95**	4.5	15.4	1.7	0.4
raspberry & redcurrant	**95**	4.5	15.4	1.7	0.5
strawberry	**97**	4.3	16.3	1.6	0.2
Vitality MÜLLER					
apple & prune	**97**	4.7	15.5	1.8	n/a
apricot	**98**	4.7	15.8	1.8	n/a
cherry	**103**	4.7	17	1.8	n/a
peach & passionfruit	**113**	4.8	19.4	1.8	n/a
pineapple	**104**	4.7	15.8	1.8	n/a
prune	**100**	4.7	16.2	1.8	n/a
raspberry	**97**	4.8	15.4	1.8	n/a
strawberry	**97**	4.7	15.8	1.8	n/a
Wild Berries Yogurt SHAPE	**46**	4.6	6.7	0.1	2.1
Wild Blueberry SVELTESSE	**53**	4.7	8.1	0.2	0.6
YOGURT DRINKS					
Benecol Yogurt Drink, each					
MCNEIL CONSUMER NUTRITIONAL	**61**	1.8	10	1.5	n/a
light	**38**	1.9	5	1.5	n/a
strawberry	**39**	2.2	4.3	1.5	n/a
Pro.active Yogurt Drinks, FLORA					
all flavours, as sold	**87**	2.6	12.5	2.9	Tr

All amounts per 100g/100ml unless otherwise stated	Cal kcal	Pro g	Carb g	Fat g	Fibre g
Vitality Drink, each MÜLLER					
cranberry	**75**	2.6	12.9	1.4	n/a
cranberry & raspberry	**43**	3.4	7.2	0.1	n/a
peach	**75**	2.6	13	1.4	n/a
raspberry	**74**	2.6	12.8	1.4	n/a
strawberry	**79**	2.6	14.1	1.4	n/a
vanilla	**75**	2.6	12.8	1.4	n/a
Yakult Fermented Milk Drink,					
each YAKULT UK	**50**	0.8	12	Tr	n/a
light, each	**30.7**	0.8	7.9	Tr	n/a

BUTTER & MARGARINES

Butter					
lightly salted ANCHOR	**740**	Tr	Tr	81.5	n/a
lightly salted LURPAK	**741**	1	1	81.5	0
lightly salted, organic YEO VALLEY	**737**	0.5	Tr	81.7	n/a
spreadable	**745**	0.5	Tr	82.5	0
spreadable LURPAK	**728**	1	1	80	0
spreadable YEO VALLEY	**720**	0.4	0.5	80	Tr
Lighter spreadable LURPAK	**544**	0.5	0.5	60	0
salted & unsalted	**744**	0.6	0.6	82.2	0
unsalted LURPAK	**749**	0	0.8	82.4	0

Margarine, hard animal &					
vegetable fat, over 80% fat	**718**	0.2	1	79.3	n/a
Stork, block STORK	**675**	0	0	75	0

All amounts per 100g/100ml unless otherwise stated	Cal kcal	Pro g	Carb g	Fat g	Fibre g
Margarine, soft					
polyunsaturated, over 80% fat	**746**	Tr	0.2	82.8	n/a
Stork, tub STORK	**531**	Tr	Tr	59	0
SPREADS					
Benecol BENECOL	**573**	0.6	1	63	0
Light	**318**	2.8	0.2	34	0
Bertolli, olive oil spread BERTOLLI	**536**	0.2	1	59	Tr
Carapelli, olive oil spread ST IVEL	**536**	0.5	0.8	59	0
Clover DAIRY CREST	**654**	0.6	0.9	72	0
Flora FLORA					
59% Vegetable Fat Spread	**531**	Tr	Tr	59	0
Buttery	**532**	Tr	0.2	59	0
Diet	**227**	3.5	1.6	23	Tr
Light	**366**	0.1	6	38	0
No Salt	**531**	Tr	Tr	59	0
Pro.active	**331**	0.1	4	35	Tr
Pro.active with olive oil	**331**	0.1	4	35	Tr
Gold ST IVEL	**330**	0.5	3.1	35	0
I Can't Believe It's Not Butter BESTFOODS	**533**	0.2	0.3	59	0
Utterly Butterly ST IVEL	**534**	0.3	0.5	59	0
Scandinavian style	**606**	0.3	0.5	67	0

All amounts per 100g/100ml unless otherwise stated	Cal kcal	Pro g	Carb g	Fat g	Fibre g
Vitalite DAIRY CREST	**503**	0	0	56	n/a
Willow DAIRY CREST	**708**	0.6	0.9	78	n/a

CHEESES

All amounts per 100g/100ml unless otherwise stated	Cal kcal	Pro g	Carb g	Fat g	Fibre g
Babybel, mini FROMAGERIES BEL	**299**	23	Tr	23	n/a
Bavarian Smoked	**277**	17	0.4	23	0
Boursin BOURSIN					
ail & fines herbs	**405**	7	2	41	Tr
au poivre	**405**	7	2	41	Tr
light	**140**	12	2.5	9	Tr
Brie	**305**	22	0.5	24	0
Caerphilly	**371**	23	0.1	31	0
Cambozola	**430**	13	0.5	42	0
Camembert	**290**	21.5	Tr	22.7	0
Cathedral City DAIRY CREST	**416**	25.4	0.1	34.9	0
Cheddar					
English	**416**	25.4	0.1	34.9	0
vegetarian	**390**	25.5	Tr	32	0
mild, organic YEO VALLEY	**410**	25	0.1	34.4	n/a
Cheddar-type, half fat	**273**	32.7	Tr	15.8	0
Cheshire	**371**	23	0.1	31	0
organic YEO VALLEY	**377**	23.5	0.1	31.4	n/a

All amounts per 100g/100ml unless otherwise stated	Cal kcal	Pro g	Carb g	Fat g	Fibre g
Cottage Cheese					
plain	**101**	12.6	3.1	4.3	0
reduced fat	**79**	13.3	3.3	1.5	0
with additions	**95**	12.8	2.6	3.8	
natural WEIGHT WATCHERS	**68**	10.3	5.7	0.4	0.2
Cracker Barrel Cheddar KRAFT	**415**	25	0.1	34.5	0
Cream Cheese	**439**	3.1	Tr	47.4	n/a
Danish Blue	**342**	20.5	Tr	28.9	0
Dolcelatte	**395**	17	0.8	36	0
Double Gloucester	**402**	24	0.1	34	0
organic YEO VALLEY	**404**	24.4	0.1	34	n/a
Edam	**341**	26.7	Tr	26	0
Emmenthal	**370**	29	0.4	28	0
Feta	**250**	15.6	1.5	20.2	0
Goats' Milk Soft Cheese	**320**	21.1	1	25.8	0
Gorgonzola	**310**	19	0	26	0
Gouda	**377**	25.3	Tr	30.6	0
Grana Padano	**392**	35	0	28	0
Gruyère	**396**	27	0.1	32	0
Jarlsberg	**364**	28	0	28	0
Lancashire	**371**	23	0.1	31	0

All amounts per 100g/100ml unless otherwise stated	Cal kcal	Pro g	Carb g	Fat g	Fibre g
Laughing Cow FROMAGERIES BEL	**269**	10	6.5	22.5	n/a
Light	**141**	13	6.5	7	n/a
Mascarpone	**416**	4.8	4.8	42	0
Mature Cheese, reduced fat WEIGHT WATCHERS	**306**	27	0.1	22	0
Medium Fat Soft Cheese	**199**	9.8	3.5	16.3	0
Mild Cheese, reduced fat WEIGHT WATCHERS	**306**	27	0.1	22	0
Mozzarella	**257**	18.6	Tr	20.3	0
Parmesan, fresh	**415**	36.2	0.9	29.7	0
Philadelphia Soft Cheese KRAFT					
Full Fat	**250**	5.9	3.2	24	0.2
Light Medium Fat	**189**	7.8	3.5	15.5	0.4
Light with chives	**185**	7.5	3.4	15.5	0.3
Light with garlic & herbs	**180**	7.2	3.4	15.5	0.2
Extra Light	**101**	11	3	5	0.6
Quark	**61**	11	3.9	0.2	0
Red Leicester	**402**	24	0.1	34	0
organic YEO VALLEY	**399**	23.8	0.1	33.7	n/a
Ricotta	**134**	9	2	10	0
Roquefort	**355**	23	Tr	29.2	0
Sage Derby	**415**	24.4	2.7	34	0

All amounts per 100g/100ml unless otherwise stated	Cal kcal	Pro g	Carb g	Fat g	Fibre g
Shropshire Blue	369	22	0.5	31	0
Soft Cheese, low fat					
WEIGHT WATCHERS	95	11.2	5.1	3.3	3
Stilton					
blue	410	23.7	0.1	35	0
white	359	20	0.1	31	0
white, with apricots	321	16	8	25	1.4
Wensleydale	380	23	0.1	32	0
with cranberries	363	21	9	27	0

CHEESE SPREADS & PROCESSED CHEESE

	Cal kcal	Pro g	Carb g	Fat g	Fibre g
Cheese Spread					
plain	267	11.3	4.4	22.8	0
reduced fat	175	15	7.9	9.5	0
WEIGHT WATCHERS	112	18.1	3.4	2.9	1.2
with roasted onion					
WEIGHT WATCHERS	123	18.1	5.8	3	0.5
Cheese Slices KRAFT					
singles	260	13.5	7.6	14.5	0.5
singles light	205	20	6	11	0
Cheestrings, all varieties					
GOLDEN VALE	328	28	Tr	24	n/a
Dairylea Cheese Food Slices,					
thick KRAFT	280	13	9.5	21	0
thick light	205	17.3	8.6	10.5	0

All amounts per 100g/100ml unless otherwise stated	Cal kcal	Pro g	Carb g	Fat g	Fibre g
Dairylea Cheese Portions KRAFT	**240**	10.5	6.1	19.5	0
Dairylea Cheese Rippers KRAFT	**260**	24.5	1.2	17	0
Dairylea Cheese Strip Cheese KRAFT	**350**	21.5	1	27.5	0
Primula PRIMULA					
original	**249**	13.8	3.6	19.9	0.5
cheese & chive	**236**	12.4	3.9	19	0.5
cheese & ham	**238**	13.3	3.5	19	0.5
cheese & shrimp	**234**	14.3	2.6	18.5	0.5
light with cracked black pepper	**137**	17.2	4.8	5.4	0.5
Processed Cheese, plain	**297**	17.8	5	23	0

See also: **SAVOURY SPREADS & PASTES**

DELI & COLD MEAT

All amounts per 100g/100ml unless otherwise stated	Cal kcal	Pro g	Carb g	Fat g	Fibre g
Beef, roasted					
silverside	**138**	19.1	2.4	5.8	Tr
topside	**158**	25	0.4	6	n/a
Chicken, roasted					
breast	**152**	27	0.2	4.8	Tr
Chorizo	**387**	23	4	31	0
Corned Beef					
canned	**205**	25.9	1	10.9	n/a
canned PRINCE'S	**223**	24.8	0.5	13.5	n/a
Garlic Sausage	**189**	15.3	5.8	11.6	0.5
coarse	**222**	22	0.9	15	0.4
Haggis, boiled	**310**	10.7	19.2	21.7	n/a
Ham & Pork, chopped, canned	**275**	14.4	1.4	23.6	0.3
Ham					
canned PRINCE'S	**164**	12	2	12	Tr
cooked, wafer thin	**98**	17	1	2.9	0
honey roast	**139**	22	3	4.3	0
honey roast, wafer thin	**104**	17	3.9	2.3	0
mustard	**123**	23	1.8	2.6	0
Parma	**240**	25	0.1	15	0
on the bone	**136**	21	0.8	6	0.7
smoked, wafer thin	**98**	17	1	2.9	0
Wiltshire	**201**	19.9	1.5	12.8	1.1
Yorkshire	**139**	21	0.3	6	0.5

All amounts per 100g/100ml unless otherwise stated	Cal kcal	Pro g	Carb g	Fat g	Fibre g
Haslet	**144**	13	19	2	0.8
Kabanos	**240**	24	1	15	0.5
Liver Pâté	**348**	12.6	0.8	32.7	n/a
reduced fat	**191**	18	3	12	Tr
Liver Sausage	**226**	13.4	6	16.7	n/a
Luncheon Meat, canned	**279**	12.9	3.6	23.8	n/a
Pâté, Brussels	**345**	12	4	31	0.2
CASTLE MACLELLAN	**329**	10.9	3.8	27.4	1.3
Peperami PEPERAMI					
Firestick	**558**	19	3.5	52	1.2
Hot	**554**	19	2.5	52	1.2
Minis	**536**	22	1.7	49	0.1
Pork Salami Sausage	**536**	22	1.7	49	0.1
Polony	**281**	9.4	14.2	21.1	n/a
Pork					
luncheon meat	**267**	14	3.3	22	0
oven-baked	**183**	26	1.4	8	0.8
roast with stuffing	**160**	18	3.3	8	1.1
stuffed pork roll TYNE BRAND	**147**	4.5	9.6	7	n/a
Salami	**438**	20.9	0.5	39.2	n/a
Danish	**604**	15.6	0.5	59.9	0
German	**395**	19	1	35	0
Milano	**428**	23	3	36	0

All amounts per 100g/100ml unless otherwise stated	Cal kcal	Pro g	Carb g	Fat g	Fibre g
Scotch Eggs	**241**	12	13.1	16	N
Tongue, lunch	**175**	19.5	0.3	10.4	0
Turkey					
breast, roasted, sliced cooked, wafer thin	**115**	25	0.6	1.4	0
BERNARD MATTHEWS	**137**	13.1	5.5	7	0.8
stuffed turkey roll TYNE BRAND	**150**	13	7.8	7.4	n/a

DESSERTS & PUDDINGS

All amounts per 100g/100ml unless otherwise stated	Cal kcal	Pro g	Carb g	Fat g	Fibre g
PUDDINGS & TRIFLES					
Bread Pudding, recipe	**289**	5.9	48	9.5	n/a
Chocolova McVITIE'S	**351**	3.4	42.3	18.7	Tr
Christmas Pudding	**329**	3	56.3	11.8	n/a
Meringue	**381**	5.3	96	Tr	n/a
Pavlova McVITIE'S					
fruits of the forest	**293**	2.7	43.6	12	Tr
raspberry	**297**	2.5	45	11.9	Tr
strawberry	**330**	2.3	32.7	21.1	0
Profiteroles McVITIE'S	**358**	6.2	18.5	29.2	0.4
Sago Pudding					
made with semi-skimmed milk	**93**	4	20.1	0.2	0.1
made with whole milk	**130**	4.1	19.6	4.3	0.1
as sold WHITWORTHS	**355**	0.2	94	0.2	0
Semolina Pudding					
made with semi-skimmed milk	**93**	4	20.1	0.2	0.1
made with whole milk	**130**	4.1	19.6	4.3	0.1
as sold WHITWORTHS	**334**	11.1	69.2	1.4	3.7
Tapioca Pudding					
made with semi-skimmed milk	**93**	4	20.1	0.2	0.1
made with whole milk	**130**	4.1	19.6	4.3	0.1
as sold WHITWORTHS	**348**	0.4	86.4	0.1	0.4
Torte, raspberry McVITIE'S	**271**	3.5	24.5	17.8	0.4

All amounts per 100g/100ml unless otherwise stated	Cal kcal	Pro g	Carb g	Fat g	Fibre g
Trifle	**166**	2.6	21	8.1	Tr
raspberry, luxury WEIGHT WATCHERS	**110**	3.2	18.4	1.8	0.4
strawberry YOUNG'S	**142**	1.4	26.6	3.7	0.2
Trifle Mixes, as sold BIRD'S					
raspberry	**420**	2.5	77	10.5	1.5
sherry flavour	**420**	2.5	77	10.5	1.5
strawberry	**420**	2.5	77	10.5	1.5
Trifle with Fresh Cream	**166**	2.4	19.5	9.2	0.5
Trifle, Luxury Devonshire ST IVEL					
fruit cocktail	**166**	2	23.3	7.2	0.2
mandarin & banana	**190**	2.4	22.5	10.1	0.1
raspberry	**167**	2.1	23.2	7.3	0.3
strawberry	**166**	2.1	23.2	7.2	0.2

SPONGE & RICE PUDDINGS

All amounts per 100g/100ml unless otherwise stated	Cal kcal	Pro g	Carb g	Fat g	Fibre g
Creamed Macaroni AMBROSIA	**90**	3.7	15	1.7	0.3
Creamed Rice Dessert Pot AMBROSIA					
as sold	**104**	3.3	17	2.5	Tr
low fat	**87**	3.3	16.5	0.9	Tr
Creamed Rice AMBROSIA	**93**	3.2	16	2.9	Tr
low fat AMBROSIA	**83**	3.2	15.7	0.8	Tr
organic AMBROSIA	**110**	3.5	15.6	3.7	Tr
strawberry WEIGHT WATCHERS	**84**	3.1	16.1	0.8	1
Traditional AMBROSIA	**107**	3.3	17	2.9	0.1
vanilla WEIGHT WATCHERS	**83**	3.2	16	0.7	0.3

All amounts per 100g/100ml unless otherwise stated	Cal kcal	Pro g	Carb g	Fat g	Fibre g
Creamed Sago AMBROSIA	**79**	2.7	13.4	1.6	0.2
Creamed Semolina AMBROSIA	**79**	3.3	12.6	1.7	0.2
Creamed Tapioca AMBROSIA	**75**	2.7	12.4	1.6	0
Müllerice MÜLLER					
apple	**122**	3.3	21.7	2.4	n/a
apple, only 1% fat	**83**	3.5	15.3	0.9	n/a
caramel	**105**	3.5	17.4	2.4	n/a
original, only 1% fat	**72**	3.9	11.8	1	n/a
raisin & nutmeg	**122**	3.3	22	2.3	n/a
raspberry	**114**	3.4	20	2.3	n/a
raspberry, only 1% fat	**77**	3.5	13.8	0.9	n/a
strawberry	**115**	3.4	20	2.4	n/a
strawberry, only 1% fat	**77**	3.5	13.6	0.9	n/a
vanilla custard	**125**	3.3	22.1	2.6	n/a
Rice Pudding					
recipe	**130**	4.1	19.6	4.3	0.1
canned	**85**	3.3	16.1	1.3	N
canned CREAMOLA	**380**	6.4	85	1	2.4
Sponge Pudding HEINZ	**340**	5.8	45.3	16.3	1.1
Banana with Toffee Sauce	**291**	2.7	48.8	9.4	0.7
Chocolate with Cadbury Chocolate Sauce	**303**	5.2	44.6	11.5	1.2
Chocolate with Chocolate Sauce	**290**	3.1	48.2	9.5	1.4
Lemon	**306**	2.7	50.1	10.6	0.6
Mixed Fruit	**302**	4	44.5	12	1.3

All amounts per 100g/100ml unless otherwise stated	Cal kcal	Pro g	Carb g	Fat g	Fibre g
Sticky Toffee	**311**	3.3	47.4	12	0.7
Strawberry Jam	**289**	3.2	51.1	8	0.6
Treacle	**286**	2.6	50	8.4	0.6
Spotted Dick HEINZ	**337**	3.4	52.7	12.6	1

CHILLED DESSERTS

Aero Chocolate Mousse NESTLÉ	**229**	4.1	27.6	11.4	1.1
Aero Milk Chocolate Mousse NESTLÉ	**185**	5.1	21	8.9	0.5
Aero Orange Mousse NESTLÉ	**218**	4.1	23.6	11.9	0.8
Aero Peppermint Mousse NESTLÉ	**218**	4.1	23.6	11.9	0.8
American Classics Corner MÜLLER					
Alabama chocolate fudge cake	**180**	3.4	27.5	6.3	n/a
blueberry Manhattan cheesecake	**152**	3.5	23.8	4.8	n/a
Florida Key Lime pie	**166**	4.4	22.6	6.4	n/a
New England banofee pie	**180**	3.6	27.7	6.1	n/a
Amoré Continental Mousses MÜLLER					
Black Cherries with Amaretto	**142**	3.4	23.2	4	n/a
Raspberry Crème	**141**	3.5	22.4	4.1	n/a
Black Cherry Ripple Mousse, each FIESTA	**87**	2	11.6	4	n/a
Cadbury Crunchie Twinpot MÜLLER	**270**	5.6	33.8	12.7	n/a

All amounts per 100g/100ml unless otherwise stated	Cal kcal	Pro g	Carb g	Fat g	Fibre g
Cadbury Flake Twinpot MÜLLER	275	6.2	29.8	14.6	n/a
Cadbury Light Mousse MÜLLER	125	6.2	17.3	3.3	n/a
Cadbury Light Orange Mousse MÜLLER	125	6.2	17.3	3.3	n/a
Cadbury Light Trifle MÜLLER	185	5.5	23.4	7.5	n/a
Cadbury Mousse MÜLLER	195	6.1	24.3	8.2	n/a
Cadbury Trifle MÜLLER	285	5.2	24.3	18.5	n/a
Caramel Soya Dessert, Alpro, each PROVAMEL	82	3	13.4	1.7	0.5
Chocolate & Vanilla Mousse WEIGHT WATCHERS	132	4.4	22.2	2.8	0.9
Chocolate Dessert, Alpro, organic PROVAMEL	87	3	13.6	2.3	1.2
Chocolate Mousse	149	4	19.9	6.5	N
WEIGHT WATCHERS	97	4.8	10.3	3.6	0.4
each FIESTA	83	1.9	10.2	3.8	n/a
Creme Brulee, raspberry & redcurrant McVITIE'S	251	1.3	23.5	17	0.2
Creme Caramel	104	3	20.6	1.6	n/a
Crunch Corner MÜLLER					
banana choco flakes	145	4.1	22.5	4.3	n/a
strawberry orange balls	145	4.1	22.5	4.3	n/a

All amounts per 100g/100ml unless otherwise stated	Cal kcal	Pro g	Carb g	Fat g	Fibre g
toffee hoops	**145**	4.1	22.5	4.3	n/a
vanilla choco balls	**145**	4.1	22.5	4.3	n/a
Dessert Corner MÜLLER					
Lemon Cheesecake	**149**	3.7	23.9	4.3	n/a
Mississippi Mud Pie	**169**	4.1	26.3	5.3	n/a
Rhubarb Crumble	**148**	3.3	21.7	5.3	n/a
Strawberry Crumble	**148**	3.3	21.7	5.3	n/a
Fruit Mousse	**143**	4.5	18	6.4	N
Healthy Balance Corner MÜLLER					
black cherry	**89**	**3.8**	**15.2**	**1.5**	n/a
pineapple, passionfruit & papaya	**87**	3.8	14.7	1.5	n/a
tropical crunch	**125**	5.3	19.7	2.8	n/a
Lemon Fruit Juice Mousse SHAPE	**76**	3.7	13.8	0.7	Tr
Lemon Moussecake WEIGHT WATCHERS	**144**	3.2	26.7	2.7	0.5
Milky Bar Dessert NESTLÉ	**266**	5	22	17.6	0.6
Mint Choc Chip Mousse, each FIESTA	**84**	1.8	10.6	4.1	n/a
Orange Fruit Juice Mousse SHAPE	**76**	3.7	13.8	0.7	Tr
Raspberry Ripple Mousse, each FIESTA	**90**	2	11.4	4	n/a
Rolo Dessert NESTLÉ	**245**	3.1	30.3	12.2	0.3

All amounts per 100g/100ml unless otherwise stated	Cal kcal	Pro g	Carb g	Fat g	Fibre g
Smatana RAINES	**130**	4.7	5.6	10	n/a
Strawberry Moussecake WEIGHT WATCHERS	**138**	3	25.5	2.7	0.5
Strawberry Fruit Juice Mousse SHAPE	**76**	3.7	13.8	0.7	Tr
Strawberry Mousse, each FIESTA	**75**	1.7	9	3.6	n/a
Tiramisu McVITIE'S	**337**	3.5	31.2	22.2	0.3
chocolate WEIGHT WATCHERS	**181**	4.1	26.9	3.7	0.8
Toffee Chocolate Dessert WEIGHT WATCHERS	**190**	5.9	32.9	3.6	0.4
Toffee Mousse, each FIESTA	**78**	1.8	9.6	3.8	n/a
Vanilla Dessert, organic, each PROVAMEL	**131**	3.8	23.9	2.3	1.3
Vanilla Soya Dessert, Alpro, each PROVAMEL	**80**	3.8	16.4	2.3	1.3

ICE CREAM & FROZEN DESSERTS

Banoffee Dessert WALLS	**107**	3.3	27.6	9.1	0.2
Caramel Ice Cream CARTE D'OR	**117**	2.4	33	7.2	0.1
Chocolate Marshmallow, Luxurious Iced Dessert WEIGHT WATCHERS	**194**	3.2	34.5	4.7	1.3

All amounts per 100g/100ml unless otherwise stated	Cal kcal	Pro g	Carb g	Fat g	Fibre g
Chocolate Brownie Dessert					
WALLS	110	3.8	25.6	9.2	1.5
Chocolate Creme de Creme,					
each LYONS MAID	161	3.2	17.5	8.8	n/a
Chocolate Ice Cream					
light CARTE D'OR	77	3.1	24	5	4.9
FIESTA	187	3.5	20.6	10.6	n/a
LYONS MAID	91	2	11.4	4.2	n/a
Chocolate Nut Sundae	243	2.6	26.2	14.9	0.1
Chocolate Ripple Ice Cream					
LYONS MAID	98	2	14.2	3.7	n/a
Chunky Choc Ice WALLS	160	3.8	24.4	16.8	0.2
Cornetto WALLS					
classic	199	2.7	37.3	11.4	1.1
mint	158	3.9	28.6	14.7	1.2
strawberry	171	2.7	37.2	11.4	1.1
whippy	188	3.6	34	16	0.7
Cornish Ice Cream LYONS MAID	92	19	11.3	4.4	n/a
Dark Classico, each LYONS MAID	135	1.5	13.5	8.5	n/a
Feast WALLS	293	3.7	27.2	27.2	1
Galaxy Bar, each MARS	184	2.1	16.6	12.2	0.3
Galaxy Caramel Swirl Ice Cream					
MARS	338	3.8	33	21.3	n/a

All amounts per 100g/100ml unless otherwise stated	Cal kcal	Pro g	Carb g	Fat g	Fibre g
Galaxy Triple Chocolate Swirls					
Ice Cream	**345**	3.9	32.7	22.1	n/a
Ice Cream: *see* **Individual flavours**					
Ice Cream Bar, chocolate coated	311	5	21.8	23.3	Tr
on a stick, organic GREEN & BLACK	233	3.7	18.5	16	1.6
Ice Cream Cone, each					
strawberry & vanilla RICHMOND	162	2.3	21.7	7.3	0.4
Ice Cream Desserts, frozen	251	3.5	21	17.6	Tr
Ice Lollies TROPICANA					
Orange 'n' Cream	128	1.4	20.5	4.5	0.3
Strawberries 'n' Cream	117	1.6	25	1.2	n/a
Triple Citrus	115	0.2	28.1	Tr	0.1
King Cone, each LYONS MAID					
Mega Mint	367	6.2	46.4	18.7	n/a
Mint Chocolate Chip	185	3	23.6	8.6	n/a
Strawberry	186	2	28.9	6.8	n/a
Vanilla	174	2.8	23.6	7.6	n/a
Lavazza Ice Cream CARTE D'OR	116	3.5	29	9.8	0.4
Lemon Meringue Dessert WALLS	100	2.6	27.1	8.2	0.2
M & Ms Ice Cream Cone MARS	321	3.8	36.8	17.6	n/a
Magnum 5 Senses WALLS					
Aroma	285	4.6	30	21	2.6
Sound	260	4.8	28	21	3.1

All amounts per 100g/100ml unless otherwise stated	Cal kcal	Pro g	Carb g	Fat g	Fibre g
Taste	**280**	4.1	31	21	0.8
Touch	**289**	4.7	30	21	1.7
Vision	**226**	3.4	33	15	0.8
Magnum 6th Sense WALLS	**266**	5.5	34	22	1.7
Magnum Almond, snack size WALLS	**190**	5	32	21	0.1
Magnum Classic WALLS	**256**	4	29	19	1.3
Snack Size	**170**	4.3	33	20	1
Magnum Light WALLS	**170**	3.8	20	12	n/a
Magnum White WALLS	**256**	4.1	30	18	0.2
Snack Size	**175**	4.3	34	20	0
Maltesers Ice Cream MARS	**253**	2.7	23.3	16.6	0.5
Mars Bar Ice Cream MARS	**346**	4.4	37.3	19.6	n/a
Marscapone Ice Cream CARTE D'OR	**120**	2.8	29	8.9	0.3
Milk Classico, each LYONS MAID	**141**	1.7	13.5	9	n/a
Mint Choc Chip Ice Cream LYONS MAID	**73**	1.2	9.7	3.3	0.1
Mint Crisp, each LYONS MAID	**198**	1.7	22	11.4	n/a
Napoli LYONS MAID					
banana	**95**	1.7	10.5	5.1	n/a
blueberry	**104**	1.8	12.7	5.2	n/a
chocolate ripple	**121**	2.3	14.9	5.9	n/a

All amounts per 100g/100ml unless otherwise stated	Cal kcal	Pro g	Carb g	Fat g	Fibre g
coffee	**98**	1.9	10.4	5.5	n/a
maple walnut	**118**	2	12.9	6.5	n/a
mint chocolate chip	**124**	2.1	13.7	6.8	n/a
rum & raisin	**104**	1.8	12.4	5.1	n/a
strawberry	**102**	1.8	12.2	5.1	n/a
toffee	**107**	1.8	14.5	5.8	n/a
vanilla	**100**	1.9	10.6	5.6	n/a
Neapolitan Ice Cream FIESTA	**173**	3.6	20.1	9.3	n/a
LYONS MAID	**83**	1.7	11.8	3.3	Tr
WALLS	**92**	2.8	23.5	8.6	0.2
Passionfruit & Mango Iced Dessert					
WEIGHT WATCHERS	**147**	1.8	29.1	2.6	0.6
Peach Melba Ice Cream					
LYONS MAID	**94**	1.7	13.2	3.8	n/a
Raspberry Ripple Ice Cream					
FIESTA	**192**	3.2	24.3	9.8	n/a
LYONS MAID	**87**	1.6	13.1	3.1	Tr
Raspberry Swirl Iced Dessert					
WEIGHT WATCHERS	**124**	1.7	23.4	2.5	0.3
Rum & Raisin Ice Cream					
LYONS MAID	**74**	1.1	10.7	2.9	0.1
Snickers Ice Cream Bar MARS	**352**	7.1	31.7	21.9	0.7
Solero WALLS					
Exotic	**100**	1.8	23.5	3.6	0.5

All amounts per 100g/100ml unless otherwise stated	Cal kcal	Pro g	Carb g	Fat g	Fibre g
Red Fruits	**100**	1.6	25.2	2.8	1.5
Orange Fresh	**75**	0.3	24.6	0	0.5
Peach Yoghurt	**108**	2	19.1	3.9	0.3
Solero Shots, Cool Lemon WALLS	**25**	0.1	3.9	1.3	n/a
Sorbet					
fruit	**97**	0.2	24.8	0.3	1
lemon	**128**	0	32	0	0
lemon FIESTA	**114**	0	28.1	0	n/a
Starburst Joosters MARS	**131**	1.2	31.4	0	n/a
Starburst MARS					
orange & lemon	**119**	0.2	29.3	0.1	n/a
strawberry	**127**	0.1	31.8	0.1	n/a
Spagnola Ice Cream CARTE D'OR	**105**	2	32.1	5.6	0.3
Strawberry Creme de Creme, each LYONS MAID	**174**	2.3	26	7.2	n/a
Strawberry Frozen Yogurt, organic YEO VALLEY	**140**	4.8	23.5	3	0.1
Strawberry Ice Cream					
CARTE D'OR	**104**	4.2	24	7.9	0.5
FIESTA	**176**	3.8	18.5	10.2	n/a
LYONS MAID	**84**	1.7	10.5	3.8	n/a
Terry's Chocolate Orange Ice Cream CARTE D'OR	**103**	2.7	27	7.2	1.3

All amounts per 100g/100ml unless otherwise stated	Cal kcal	Pro g	Carb g	Fat g	Fibre g
Triple Chocolate Ice Cream					
CARTE D'OR	**116**	3.5	27	9.9	1.3
LYONS MAID	**77**	1.3	11.4	2.9	0.1
Toblerone Ice Cream CARTE D'OR	**119**	3.8	29	9.3	1.1
Toffee Crumble, each LYONS MAID	**170**	1.9	19.6	9.3	n/a
Toffee Flavour & Toffee Sauce Iced Dessert WEIGHT WATCHERS	**163**	2.7	26.2	4.8	0.2
Toffee Flavour Fudge Swirl Iced Dessert WEIGHT WATCHERS	**143**	2.5	22.6	4.4	0.4
Tornado, each LYONS MAID	**61**	0	15.2	0	n/a
Tropical Juice Bar, each LYONS MAID	**37**	Tr	9.9	Tr	n/a
Twix Ice Cream MARS	**400**	5.4	43	22.9	n/a
Vanilla & Raspberry Compote Iced Dessert WEIGHT WATCHERS	**142**	2.6	23.3	3.9	0.3
Vanilla & Strawberry Compote Iced Dessert WEIGHT WATCHERS	**142**	2.5	23.4	3.9	0.2
Vanilla Creme de Creme, each LYONS MAID	**166**	3	21.3	8.3	n/a
Vanilla Cup, each LYONS MAID	**181**	3.3	25.5	8.1	n/a
Vanilla Ice Cream CARTE D'OR	**102**	3	26	9.1	0.2
FIESTA	**155**	3.6	19.2	7.6	n/a
LYONS MAID	**87**	1.7	11	4.5	n/a

All amounts per 100g/100ml unless otherwise stated	Cal kcal	Pro g	Carb g	Fat g	Fibre g
Cream of Cornish WALLS	**89**	3.5	22.5	8.9	0.1
light CARTE D'OR	**66**	2.2	21	4.4	4
organic YEO VALLEY	**209**	5.1	21.8	11.3	0
soft scoop WALLS	**83**	2.9	23.5	9.1	0.2
soft serve FIESTA	**161**	3.3	19.4	8.3	n/a
super value FIESTA	**154**	3.4	20.4	7.1	n/a
Vanilla Iced Dessert					
WEIGHT WATCHERS	**124**	2.4	20.1	3.5	0.2
Viennetta WALLS					
biscuit forest fruit	**143**	3.3	27.6	15.8	0.6
brownie	**145**	4.2	28.4	15.5	0.9
chocolate	**123**	4.1	22.2	16.6	1.6
double crisp	**144**	3.7	24.9	16.9	0.9
mint	**125**	3.3	22.3	16.9	0.3
strawberry	**127**	3.4	23	16.9	0.3
vanilla	**124**	3.3	21.8	16.8	0.3

See also: **KIDS' FOODS**

CHEESECAKES

Blackcurrant Cheesecake

BONNE BOUCHE	**270**	3.4	40.1	10.7	0.4
EDEN VALE	**261**	2.8	38.8	11.6	n/a
MCVITIE'S	**296**	4.5	31.9	17.1	0.7
SARA LEE	**275**	3.4	35.1	13.4	1.4
WEIGHT WATCHERS	**159**	6	24	4.1	0.7

All amounts per 100g/100ml unless otherwise stated	Cal kcal	Pro g	Carb g	Fat g	Fibre g
Blackcurrant Party Cheesecake					
McVitie's	**295**	4.4	33.8	16.1	0.8
Cheesecake, frozen	**294**	4	35.2	16.2	1
Cherry Cream Cheesecake					
McVitie's	**336**	4.9	30	22	1.4
Chocolate Truffle Cheesecake					
McVitie's	**340**	5.9	35.4	19.7	0.6
Fruits of the Forest Cheesecake					
McVitie's	**302**	4.5	31.9	17.7	0.6
Raspberry Cheesecake Young's	**299**	4.7	31.9	17.2	0.6
Strawberry Cheesecake					
McVitie's	**390**	4.9	31.9	22.7	0.4
Sara Lee	**272**	3.1	35.3	13.2	1
Weight Watchers	**179**	5	32.6	3.2	2.8
Strawberry & Cream Cheesecake					
Young's	**296**	4.6	31.9	16.9	0.2

See also: **FLOUR & BAKING**

JELLY

Blackcurrant Flavour Jelly Crystals, sugar free Bird's	**330**	57.5	13	0.1	0
Jelly, made with water, all varieties	**61**	1.2	15.1	0	n/a

All amounts per 100g/100ml unless otherwise stated	Cal kcal	Pro g	Carb g	Fat g	Fibre g
Jelly, table,					
all varieties CHIVERS	**296**	5.1	68.9	0	n/a
all varieties HARTLEY'S	**296**	4.4	69.6	0	n/a
Jelly Pots, ready to eat HARTLEY'S					
all flavours	**100**	0	25	0	n/a
low sugar, all flavours	**9**	0	2.3	0	n/a
Lemon Flavour Jelly Crystals,					
as sold DIETADE	**7**	1.5	0.1	0	0
Orange Flavour Jelly Crystals					
as sold DIETADE	**7**	1.5	0.1	0	0
sugar free, as sold BIRD'S	**335**	62.5	6.4	1.9	0
Raspberry Flavour Jelly Crystals,					
as sold DIETADE	**8**	1.6	0.2	0	0
Raspberry Flavour Jelly,					
sugar free BIRD'S	**325**	57	12.5	0.1	0.7
Strawberry Flavour Jelly Crystals,					
as sold DIETADE	**7**	1.5	0.1	0	0
Strawberry Flavour Jelly,					
sugar free BIRD'S	**325**	57.5	11.5	0.2	0.2

DESSERT POWDERS

Instant Dessert Powder					
as sold	**391**	2.4	60.1	17.3	n/a
made up with whole milk	**111**	3.1	14.8	6.3	0.2

All amounts per 100g/100ml unless otherwise stated	Cal kcal	Pro g	Carb g	Fat g	Fibre g
Angel Delight, as sold BIRD'S					
banana	**490**	2.5	72	21	0
butterscotch	**475**	2.4	73.5	19	0
butterscotch, no added sugar	**480**	4.5	61	24	0
chocolate	**455**	3.7	69.5	18	0.4
chocolate, no added sugar	**450**	6.3	56.5	22	0.6
raspberry	**490**	2.5	72	21	0
strawberry	**485**	2.5	71	21	0
strawberry, no added sugar	**490**	4.8	59	26.5	0
Blancmange Powder, as sold					
chocolate BROWN & POLSON	**339**	2.7	78	1.7	0.8
strawberry PEARCE DUFF	**100**	2.9	14.4	3.6	n/a
vanilla BROWN & POLSON	**341**	0.6	83	0.7	n/a

CUSTARD DESSERTS

Custard Dessert Pot AMBROSIA					
banana flavour	**102**	2.8	16.5	2.8	0
chocolate flavour	**114**	3.2	18.5	3	0
strawberry flavour	**102**	2.8	16.4	2.8	0
toffee flavour	**104**	2.8	16.8	2.8	0
vanilla flavour	**102**	2.8	16.4	2.8	0
Devon Custard Dessert Pot AMBROSIA					
as sold	**102**	2.9	16	2.9	0
low fat	**70**	3.1	11.9	1.1	Tr

All amounts per 100g/100ml unless otherwise stated	Cal kcal	Pro g	Carb g	Fat g	Fibre g
SWEET SAUCES & TOPPINGS					
Angel Delight Topples BIRD'S					
chocolate	**465**	5	67	20	0.5
strawberry	**450**	2.8	74.5	14	0.7
Brandy Flavour Sauce Mix,					
as sold BIRD'S	**415**	6.1	76.5	9.5	0
Brandy Sauce, ready to serve,					
as sold BIRD'S	**97**	2.7	16.5	1.5	0
Chocolate Custard Mix, as sold BIRD'S					
chocolate flavour	**415**	5.9	78.5	8.8	0.1
low fat	**405**	4.3	78.5	8.2	0
Chocolate Custard Pot AMBROSIA	**114**	3.2	18.5	3	0.1
Custard					
canned	**100**	3	14	4	Tr
made up with skimmed milk	**79**	3.8	16.8	0.1	Tr
made up with whole milk	**118**	3.9	16.2	4.5	n/a
ready to serve	**101**	2.8	16	2.9	0
dairy free, ready to serve					
PROVAMEL	**81**	3	13.3	1.8	0.3
powder, as sold CREAMOLA	**350**	0.4	92	0.7	n/a
Custard Complete Mix ROWNTREE	**412**	4.2	77.8	10.2	n/a
Custard, Original BIRD'S					
powder, as sold	**355**	0.4	87	0.5	0
ready to serve	**102**	2.8	15.5	3	0

All amounts per 100g/100ml unless otherwise stated	Cal kcal	Pro g	Carb g	Fat g	Fibre g
Devon Custard, canned AMBROSIA	102	2.9	16	2.9	0
low fat	70	3.1	11.9	1.1	0
Dream Topping, as sold BIRD'S	690	6.7	32.5	58.5	0.5
sugar free	695	7.3	30.5	60.5	0.5
Maple Syrup, organic MERIDIAN FOODS LTD	344	Tr	85.3	0.3	Tr
Rum Flavour Sauce Mix, as sold BIRD'S	415	6.1	76.5	9.5	0
Rum Sauce, ready to serve, as sold BIRD'S	91	2.8	15.5	1.5	0
Saucy Syrup TATE & LYLE					
chocolate flavour	305	1	74	0.5	0
maple flavour	306	Tr	76.5	0	0
strawberry flavour	308	Tr	77.5	0	0
toffee flavour	306	Tr	76.5	0	0
Tip Top NESTLÉ	113	4.8	9	6.3	0
squirty	276	2.4	8	26	Tr
Treat SILVER SPOON					
Dark chocolate	319	n/a	n/a	0.1	n/a
Maple	308	n/a	n/a	0.1	n/a
Milk chocolate	375	n/a	n/a	11.5	n/a
Monster Crackin'	612	n/a	n/a	45.5	n/a
Strawberry	309	n/a	n/a	0.1	n/a
Toffee	319	n/a	n/a	0.1	n/a

All amounts per 100g/100ml unless otherwise stated	Cal kcal	Pro g	Carb g	Fat g	Fibre g
White Sauce, sweet, recipe					
made with semi-skimmed milk	**152**	4	18.5	7.4	n/a
made with whole milk	**171**	3.9	18.3	9.5	n/a

DIPS & PRE-DRESSED SALADS

All amounts per 100g/100ml unless otherwise stated	Cal kcal	Pro g	Carb g	Fat g	Fibre g
Bacon Dipper WEIGHT WATCHERS	**196**	16	24	4.2	1.4
BBQ Salsa Dip WEIGHT WATCHERS	**36**	1.1	7.6	0.1	2.3
Beetroot Salad	**52**	1.1	11	0.4	2.3
Cheese & Onion Dipper					
WEIGHT WATCHERS	**196**	16	24	4.2	1.4
Coleslaw	**181**	0.9	6	17	1.8
HEINZ	**135**	1.6	9.4	10.2	1.2
with cheese	**165**	3.3	6	14	1.1
with prawns	**158**	2	6	14	1.6
Coronation Chicken	**364**	16.6	3.2	31.7	n/a
Dairylea Chipsticks Dunkers, each KRAFT					
jumbo munch	**150**	3.6	13.5	9.2	0.6
salt & vinegar	**155**	3.5	12	10.5	0.6
Dairylea Double Dunkers, each KRAFT					
Mexican	**185**	3.9	19	10	0.9
pizza	**180**	4.7	17	10	1.2
Dairylea Dunkers Breadstick KRAFT	**235**	10.5	28	8.6	0.9
Dairylea Dunkers Jumbo Tubes KRAFT	**255**	9.2	26	12.5	0.8

All amounts per 100g/100ml unless otherwise stated	Cal kcal	Pro g	Carb g	Fat g	Fibre g
Dairylea Pizza Baguette Dunkers,					
each KRAFT	160	4.4	11.8	10.6	0.7
Doritos Dippas Mexican Dips WALKERS					
extra hot salsa	40	0.9	8.5	0.2	2.2
hot salsa	40	0.9	8.5	0.2	2.2
mild salsa	40	0.9	8.5	0.2	2.2
red pepper & tomato salsa	70	1	8.4	3.6	0.5
Florida Salad	201	0.7	11	17	1.5
Guacamole Dip DISCOVERY FOODS	140	n/a	8.6	12.2	n/a
Hummus	187	7.6	11.6	12.6	n/a
Mango Salsa Dip WEIGHT WATCHERS	85	1	19.9	0.2	2.6
Mixed Pepper Salsa PRIMULA	41	1.3	8.4	0.2	0.5
Onion & Chive Dip PRIMULA	283	4.6	5.6	26.9	0.5
Pasta Salad					
chicken caesar pasta salad	179	8	21	7	1.5
pasta & cheese	255	6	15	19	1.2
pasta, honey & mustard chicken	155	7	27	2.1	2.3
pasta, mushroom & pesto	117	3.3	20	2.6	2.2
pasta, tiger prawn & tomato	125	4.6	20	2.9	2
pasta, vine ripened tomato & mozzarella	210	6	24	10	2.3
Philadelphia Dip Plain & Ciabatta Baguette Crackers, each KRAFT	118	4	8.3	7.6	1

All amounts per 100g/100ml unless otherwise stated	Cal kcal	Pro g	Carb g	Fat g	Fibre g
Philadelphia Dip Plain & Smokey Bacon Baguette Crackers, each KRAFT	115	3.8	7.3	7	1
Potato Salad	97	2	11	5	1.6
HEINZ	141	1.4	14.8	8.5	0.8
Rice Salad					
savoury rice	94	1.7	21	0.3	0.9
vegetable	143	2.1	23	4.9	0.4
Roasted Garlic & Herb Dip					
PRIMULA	299	4.1	3.5	29.8	1.9
Salsa					
Cheese OLD EL PASO	143	2.5	9.3	10.7	n/a
Chunky OLD EL PASO	32	1.2	6.6	0.1	n/a
Cool, organic MERIDIAN FOODS LTD	141	1.1	6.3	0.4	1.2
Hot MERIDIAN FOODS LTD	24	1	4.8	0.1	1.1
hot, original OLD EL PASO	31.6	1.2	6	0.3	n/a
Hot, Ranch-Style DISCOVERY FOODS	37	n/a	8.5	0.5	n/a
Medium, Ranch-Style DISCOVERY FOODS	37	n/a	8.5	0.5	n/a
mild, original OLD EL PASO	31.6	1.2	6	0.3	n/a
organic KETTLE FOODS	39	1.7	8	Tr	n/a
Picante, Thick 'n Chunky OLD EL PASO	28	1.4	4.6	0.5	n/a
Sweet Red Pepper with Sun Dried Tomato KETTLE FOODS	39	1.7	8	Tr	n/a

All amounts per 100g/100ml unless otherwise stated	Cal kcal	Pro g	Carb g	Fat g	Fibre g
Sour Cream & Chive Dip PRIMULA	**330**	4.5	2.9	33.4	0.5
Sour Cream Based Dips	**360**	2.9	4	37	n/a
Spicy Cheese Dip PRIMULA	**298**	4.8	3.2	29.6	0.5
Taramosalata	**504**	3.2	4.1	52.9	n/a
Tzatziki	**66**	3.8	1.9	4.9	n/a
Vegetable Salad HEINZ	**133**	1.5	12.6	8.5	1.3

DRIED FRUIT, NUTS & SEEDS

All amounts per 100g/100ml unless otherwise stated	Cal kcal	Pro g	Carb g	Fat g	Fibre g
DRIED FRUIT					
Apple Rings, dried					
HOLLAND & BARRETT	**238**	2	60.1	0.5	9.7
Apricots, ready to eat	**158**	4	36.5	0.6	n/a
Banana, dried, ready to eat					
HOLLAND & BARRETT	**221**	3.1	53.7	0.8	9.5
Banana Chips, dried					
HOLLAND & BARRETT	**532**	1.7	64.6	29.6	7.8
WHITWORTHS	**526**	1	59.9	31.4	1.7
Currants, dried	**267**	2.3	67.8	0.4	n/a
HOLLAND & BARRETT	**313**	2.6	75	0.4	1.9
Dates, flesh & skin, dried	**270**	3.3	68	0.2	n/a
Figs, dried	**227**	3.6	52.9	1.6	n/a
Fruit Pockets, each JORDANS					
chunky fruits & nuts	**183**	3.3	16.7	11.5	2.1
cranberry, fruit & nuts	**170**	2.8	19.7	8.9	2.3
exotic mix	**152**	05	27.8	4.4	2.1
Fruit Salad, dried					
HOLLAND & BARRETT	**184**	3.1	44.5	0.6	7.3
WHITWORTHS	**145**	2.6	39.9	0.5	4.2
Mixed Fruit, dried	**268**	2.3	68.1	0.4	n/a
Pineapple, diced & dried					
HOLLAND & BARRETT	**347**	0.1	84.1	Tr	3.4

All amounts per 100g/100ml unless otherwise stated	Cal kcal	Pro g	Carb g	Fat g	Fibre g
Prunes					
canned in juice	**79**	0.7	19.7	0.2	n/a
canned in syrup	**90**	0.6	23	0.2	n/a
ready to eat, pitted					
HOLLAND & BARRETT	**160**	2.8	38.4	0.5	6.5
ready to eat, stone in	**141**	2.5	34	0.4	5.7
Raisins, seedless	**272**	2.1	69.3	0.4	n/a
HOLLAND & BARRETT	**289**	2.1	69.3	0.4	2
WHITWORTHS	**289**	2.1	69.3	0.4	2
Sultanas	**275**	2.7	69.4	0.4	n/a
HOLLAND & BARRETT	**275**	2.7	69.4	0.4	2

NUTS & SEEDS

	Cal kcal	Pro g	Carb g	Fat g	Fibre g
Almonds					
weighed with shells	**229**	7.8	2.5	20.6	4.8
raw mixed, unblanched	**594**	20	7	54	10
flaked/ground	**632**	25	7	56	7
whole HOLLAND & BARRETT	**630**	25.4	6.5	55.8	7.4
Brazils					
weighed with shells	**314**	6.5	1.4	31.4	3.7
kernel only	**680**	14	3.1	68	5
whole HOLLAND & BARRETT	**682**	14.1	3.1	68.2	4.3
Cashews					
kernel only	**576**	18	18	48	3.2
whole nuts HOLLAND & BARRETT	**573**	17.7	18.2	48.2	9.5

All amounts per 100g/100ml unless otherwise stated	Cal kcal	Pro g	Carb g	Fat g	Fibre g
Chestnuts, kernel only	**170**	2	36.6	2.7	n/a
Coconut: see **FRUIT & VEGETABLES**					
Hazelnuts					
weighed with shell	**247**	5.4	2.3	24.1	2.5
kernel only	**668**	17	6	64	6
Hickory Nuts: see **Pecan Nuts**					
Mixed Nuts	**607**	22.9	7.9	54.1	n/a
HOLLAND & BARRETT	**623**	20.1	7.6	57.2	5.6
Monkey Nuts: see **Peanuts**					
Peanuts					
plain, weighed with shells	**389**	17.7	8.6	31.8	4.3
plain, kernel only	**564**	25.8	12.5	46	N
paleskin HOLLAND & BARRETT	**564**	25.6	12.5	46.1	6.2
Peanuts, salted: see **CRISPS & NIBBLES**					
Pecans, kernel only	**698**	11	6	70	4.7
Pine Nuts, kernel only	**688**	14	4	68.6	n/a
HOLLAND & BARRETT	**688**	14	4	68.6	1.9
Pistachios	**620**	21	8	56	6
Pistachios, salted: see **CRISPS & NIBBLES**					
Poppy Seeds	**556**	20.6	19	44	0
Pumpkin Seeds					
HOLLAND & BARRETT	**569**	24.4	15.2	45.6	5.3

All amounts per 100g/100ml unless otherwise stated	Cal kcal	Pro g	Carb g	Fat g	Fibre g
Sunflower Seeds					
HOLLAND & BARRETT	**581**	19.8	18.6	47.5	6
Walnuts					
weighed with shell	**295**	6.3	1.4	29.4	1.5
halves HOLLAND & BARRETT	**688**	14.7	3.3	68.5	3.5
halves WHITWORTHS	**525**	10.6	5	51.5	5.2

DRINKS (ALCOHOLIC)

All amounts per 100g/100ml unless otherwise stated	Cal kcal	Pro g	Carb g	Fat g	Fibre g
Advocaat	**272**	4.7	28.4	6.3	0
Bols	**257**	3.4	27	5.6	0
Bailey's Irish Cream	**320**	n/a	n/a	n/a	n/a
Beer, bitter					
best/premium	**33**	0.3	2.2	Tr	n/a
average	**30**	0.3	2.2	Tr	n/a
canned	**32**	0.3	2.3	Tr	0
draught	**32**	0.3	2.3	Tr	0
keg	**31**	0.3	2.3	Tr	0
Beer, mild, draught	**25**	0.2	1.6	Tr	0
Brandy	**222**	Tr	Tr	0	0
Breezer, each BACARDI					
cranberry	**154**	n/a	n/a	n/a	n/a
crisp apple, half sugar	**121.5**	n/a	n/a	n/a	n/a
lemon, half sugar	**121**	n/a	n/a	n/a	n/a
lime	**181**	n/a	n/a	n/a	n/a
orange	**178.8**	n/a	n/a	n/a	n/a
pineapple	**170.5**	n/a	n/a	n/a	n/a
refreshing raspberry, half sugar	**122.1**	n/a	n/a	n/a	n/a
watermelon	**151**	n/a	n/a	n/a	n/a
Brown Ale					
bottled	**30**	0.3	3	Tr	n/a
Newcastle, per bottle					
SCOTTISH & NEWCASTLE	**165**	n/a	n/a	n/a	n/a

All amounts per 100g/100ml unless otherwise stated	Cal kcal	Pro g	Carb g	Fat g	Fibre g
Cherry Brandy	**255**	Tr	32.6	0	0
Cider					
dry	**36**	Tr	2.6	0	n/a
sweet	**42**	Tr	4.3	0	n/a
vintage	**101**	Tr	7.3	0	n/a
Cider, bottle/can H P BULMER					
Scrumpy Jack	**45**	n/a	2.64	n/a	n/a
Strongbow	**36**	n/a	1.47	n/a	n/a
Woodpecker	**30**	n/a	2.38	n/a	n/a
Cognac, Courvoisier	**350**	n/a	n/a	n/a	n/a
Cointreau	**340**	n/a	n/a	n/a	n/a
Curacao	**311**	Tr	28.3	0	0
Gin	**222**	Tr	Tr	0	0
Grand Marnier	**320**	n/a	n/a	n/a	n/a
Lager					
bottled	**29**	0.2	1.5	Tr	0
French 2.8%, per 25 cl bottle	**26**	0.6	6	0	0
French 5%, per 25 cl bottle	**35**	0.7	8	0	0
per bottle HEINEKEN	**85**	n/a	n/a	n/a	n/a
per can TENNENT'S	**140**	n/a	n/a	n/a	n/a
Pale Ale, bottled	**28**	0.3	2	Tr	n/a
Port	**157**	0.1	12	0	n/a
Cockburn	**151**	n/a	n/a	n/a	n/a

All amounts per 100g/100ml unless otherwise stated	Cal kcal	Pro g	Carb g	Fat g	Fibre g
Rum	**222**	Tr	Tr	0	0
Carta Blanca BACARDI	**210**	n/a	n/a	n/a	n/a
Sherry					
dry	**116**	0.2	1.4	0	n/a
medium	**116**	0.1	5.9	0	n/a
sweet	**136**	0.3	6.9	0	n/a
Sherry HARVEY					
Bristol Cream	**154**	n/a	n/a	n/a	n/a
Club Classic	**115**	n/a	n/a	n/a	n/a
Stout					
bottled	**37**	0.3	4.2	Tr	0
extra	**39**	0.3	2.1	Tr	0
Strong Ale	**72**	0.7	6.1	Tr	0
Tia Lusso	**251**	n/a	n/a	n/a	n/a
Tia Maria	**262**	n/a	n/a	n/a	n/a
Vermouth					
dry	**109**	0.1	3	0	n/a
sweet	**151**	Tr	15.9	0	n/a
Martini Bianco BACARDI	**145**	n/a	n/a	n/a	n/a
Martini Extra Dry BACARDI	**95**	n/a	n/a	n/a	n/a
Martini Rosso BACARDI	**140**	n/a	n/a	n/a	n/a
Vintage Cider: *see* **Cider**					
Vodka	**222**	Tr	Tr	0	0

All amounts per 100g/100ml unless otherwise stated	Cal kcal	Pro g	Carb g	Fat g	Fibre g
Whisky	**222**	Tr	Tr	0	0
Laphroaig, single malt	**222**	n/a	n/a	n/a	n/a
Teacher's, blended	**222**	n/a	n/a	n/a	n/a
Wine					
red	**68**	0.1	0.2	0	n/a
rosé	**71**	0.1	2.5	0	n/a
white, dry	**66**	0.1	0.6	0	n/a
white, medium	**74**	0.1	3	0	n/a
white, sparkling	**74**	0.3	5.1	0	n/a
white, sweet	**94**	0.2	5.9	0	n/a

DRINKS (NON-ALCOHOLIC)

All amounts per 100g/100ml unless otherwise stated	Cal kcal	Pro g	Carb g	Fat g	Fibre g
JUICES & CORDIALS					
Apple 'C' LIBBY	**47**	Tr	11.7	Tr	0
Apple Crush JUSODA	**31**	n/a	9.5	Tr	Tr
Apple Fruit Juice Concentrate, organic MERIDIAN FOODS LTD	**308**	0.8	76.1	Tr	0
Apple Juice, unsweetened	**38**	0.1	9.9	0.1	n/a
DEL MONTE	**47**	0.3	10.8	Tr	n/a
cloudy COPELLA	**44**	0.4	10.3	0.1	n/a
cloudy DEL MONTE	**46**	0.1	10.7	Tr	n/a
English CAWSTON VALE	**42**	0.1	10.8	Tr	n/a
Apple Juice Drink					
BRITVIC 55	**46.1**	0.1	11	Tr	n/a
High Juice ROBINSONS	**210.1**	Tr	50.9	Tr	n/a
Apple, Cherry & Raspberry Drink ROBINSONS	**195.5**	0.2	47.6	Tr	n/a
Apple, Raspberry & Cranberry Juice Drink BRITVIC 55	**39.8**	0.1	9.4	Tr	n/a
Apple, Red Grape & Blueberry DEL MONTE	**50**	0.6	11.5	Tr	n/a
Apple & Blackberry Juice COPELLA	**42**	0.4	9.7	0.1	n/a
Apple & Blackcurrant Drink QUOSH	**72**	Tr	16.6	Tr	n/a

All amounts per 100g/100ml unless otherwise stated	Cal kcal	Pro g	Carb g	Fat g	Fibre g
ROBINSONS	**43.1**	Tr	9.7	Tr	n/a
no added sugar ROBINSONS	**8.5**	0.1	1.1	Tr	n/a
Apple & Blackcurrant Fruit Juice					
Concentrate MERIDIAN FOODS LTD	**298**	Tr	74.6	Tr	0
Apple & Cranberry Fruit Spring					
Drink ROBINSONS	**39.1**	Tr	9.3	Tr	n/a
Apple & Elderflower Cordial					
BOTTLE GREEN	**23**	0	5.6	0	0
Apple & Elderflower Juice					
COPELLA	**43**	0.4	10.2	0.1	n/a
Apple & Lime Fruit Spring					
Drink ROBINSONS	**40.2**	Tr	9.6	Tr	n/a
Apple & Mango Juice COPELLA	**43**	0.4	10.1	0.1	n/a
DEL MONTE	**48**	0.6	10.9	Tr	n/a
Apple & Mango Juice Drink,					
J2O BRITVIC	**48**	0.1	11.3	Tr	n/a
Apple & Melon Juice Drink,					
J2O BRITVIC	**43.1**	Tr	10.2	Tr	n/a
Apple & Raspberry Juice COPELLA	**41**	0.5	9.4	0.1	n/a
Apple & Raspberry Juice Drink,					
J2O BRITVIC	**53.4**	0.1	12.5	Tr	n/a
Apple & Sour Cherry Juice					
CAWSTON VALE	**44**	0.1	10.8	Tr	n/a

All amounts per 100g/100ml unless otherwise stated	Cal kcal	Pro g	Carb g	Fat g	Fibre g
Barley Water ROBINSONS					
Lemon, original	**96.5**	0.3	21.8	Tr	Tr
Orange, original	**97.4**	0.3	23.1	Tr	Tr
Blackcurrant 'C' LIBBY	**54**	Tr	13.5	Tr	0
Blackcurrant Cordial, undiluted					
BRITVIC	**56.9**	Tr	13.1	0	n/a
Blood Orange High Juice Drink					
ROBINSONS	**216.9**	0.3	52.4	Tr	n/a
Blood Orange World Fruit Drink					
DEL MONTE	**49**	0.1	12	Tr	n/a
Breakfast Juice DEL MONTE	**43**	0.6	9.6	Tr	n/a
Caribbean Fruit Burst DEL MONTE	**39**	0.1	9.5	Tr	n/a
Carrot Juice	**24**	0.5	5.7	0.1	N
Cranberry Juice Drink					
classic OCEAN SPRAY	**49**	Tr	11.7	Tr	Tr
light	**24**	0	5.5	Tr	Tr
white	**61**	0	14.9	Tr	0
Dandelion & Burdock Cordial					
BOTTLE GREEN	**26.5**	Tr	6.6	Tr	0
Elderflower Cordial BOTTLE GREEN	**23**	0	5.6	0	0
English Summer Cordial					
BOTTLE GREEN	**27**	0	6.7	0	0

All amounts per 100g/100ml unless otherwise stated	Cal kcal	Pro g	Carb g	Fat g	Fibre g
Five Alive COCA-COLA					
Berry Blast	**53**	0	13	0	n/a
Citrus Burst	**50**	Tr	12.8	0	n/a
Cranberry Splash	**37**	Tr	9.5	0	n/a
Five Alive Tropical Hit Squash					
COCA-COLA	**3**	0	0.4	0	n/a
Five Fruit 'C' LIBBY	**40**	0.1	10	Tr	Tr
Five Fruits Fruit Burst DEL MONTE	**53**	0.2	12.4	Tr	n/a
Fruit & Barley ROBINSONS					
apple & blackcurrant	**14.4**	0.2	2.2	Tr	n/a
citrus	**12.7**	0.2	1.2	Tr	n/a
orange	**16**	0.3	2.6	Tr	n/a
peach	**13.9**	0.3	2	Tr	n/a
pink grapefruit	**15.3**	0.3	2	Tr	n/a
strawberry & kiwi	**14.4**	0.2	2.2	Tr	n/a
summer fruits	**14.6**	0.2	2.3	Tr	n/a
Ginger & Lemongrass Cordial					
BOTTLE GREEN	**22**	0	5.1	0	0
Grape & Melon Soft Drink					
ROBINSONS	**216.7**	0.2	52.5	Tr	n/a
Grape Juice					
unsweetened	**46**	0.3	11.7	0.1	0
unsweetened, red, sparkling					
SCHLOER	**49**	Tr	13.1	n/a	n/a
unsweetened, white SCHLOER	**48**	Tr	12.9	n/a	n/a

All amounts per 100g/100ml unless otherwise stated	Cal kcal	Pro g	Carb g	Fat g	Fibre g
unsweetened, white, sparkling					
SCHLOER	**49**	Tr	13.1	n/a	n/a
unsweetened	**33**	0.4	8.3	0.1	Tr
BRITVIC	**39.6**	0.5	8.1	0.1	n/a
Grapefruit 'C' LIBBY	**36**	0.2	8.8	Tr	0.3
Grapefruit Fruit Juice DEL MONTE	**41**	0.5	8.8	Tr	n/a
Kiwi World Fruits Juice Drink DEL MONTE	**50**	0.2	11.9	Tr	n/a
Lemon & Lime Drink JUSODA	**28**	n/a	6.9	Tr	Tr
Lemon Drink CITRUS SPRING	**40.9**	Tr	9.6	Tr	n/a
Lemon Fruit Squash ROBINSONS	**58.4**	0.2	21.2	Tr	n/a
Lemon Low Calorie Squash DIETADE	**7**	0	0.4	0	n/a
Lemon Refresher Soft Drink, organic BRITVIC	**49.4**	Tr	11.6	Tr	n/a
Lemon Soft Drink, no added sugar ROBINSONS	**10.8**	0.2	0.4	Tr	n/a
Lemonade, All Juice CAWSTON VALE	**44**	Tr	11.7	Tr	n/a
Lime Cordial, undiluted ROSES	**104.5**	0.1	24.1	0	n/a
Lime Drink CITRUS SPRING	**45.2**	Tr	10.5	Tr	n/a
Lime Juice Cordial					
undiluted	**112**	0.1	29.8	0	n/a
undiluted BRITVIC	**46.1**	0.1	9.1	Tr	n/a

All amounts per 100g/100ml unless otherwise stated	Cal kcal	Pro g	Carb g	Fat g	Fibre g
Mango & Papaya World Fruits					
Juice Drink DEL MONTE	**63**	0.2	15.3	Tr	n/a
Orange & Cranberry Juice					
Drink, J2O BRITVIC	**48.7**	0.2	11.2	Tr	n/a
Orange & Mango Soft Drink,					
no added sugar ROBINSONS	**8.2**	0.2	0.8	Tr	n/a
Orange & Passionfruit Juice					
Drink, J2O BRITVIC	**50.4**	0.5	11.3	Tr	n/a
Orange & Pineapple Squash					
ROBINSONS	**53.2**	0.1	12.1	Tr	n/a
as sold QUOSH	**55**	0.1	12.4	Tr	n/a
no added sugar ROBINSONS	**8.7**	0.2	0.9	Tr	n/a
Orange & Pineapple Fruit Juice					
DEL MONTE	**48**	0.5	11	Tr	n/a
Orange 'C' LIBBY	**37**	0.1	9.1	Tr	0.1
no added sugar	**12**	0.2	1.9	Tr	Tr
Orange Apple Passionfruit Juice					
DEL MONTE	**45**	0.5	10.1	Tr	n/a
Orange Drink					
undiluted	**107**	Tr	28.5	0	0
CITRUS SPRING	**41.2**	Tr	9.9	Tr	n/a
JUSODA	**31**	n/a	7.6	Tr	Tr
QUOSH	**40**	0.1	8.8	Tr	n/a
Orange Fruit Burst DEL MONTE	**49**	0.1	12	Tr	n/a

All amounts per 100g/100ml unless otherwise stated	Cal kcal	Pro g	Carb g	Fat g	Fibre g
Orange Fruit Juice DEL MONTE	44	0.6	9.9	Tr	n/a
Orange Juice					
unsweetened	36	0.5	8.8	0.1	n/a
BRITVIC	45.2	0.5	9.8	0.1	n/a
CAWSTON VALE	43	0.6	10.5	Tr	n/a
Orange Juice Drink BRITVIC 55	48.9	0.3	11.3	Tr	n/a
Orange Peach Apricot Juice DEL MONTE	44	0.6	9.9	Tr	n/a
Orange Squash, undiluted					
BRITVIC	53.9	0.2	11.6	Tr	n/a
ROBINSONS	53.4	0.1	12.3	Tr	n/a
High Juice ROBINSONS	182.4	0.1	43.6	0.1	n/a
low calorie DIETADE	12	0	2.4	Tr	n/a
no added sugar ROBINSONS	7.8	0.2	0.7	Tr	n/a
Passionfruit World Fruits Juice Drink DEL MONTE	49	0.3	11.7	Tr	n/a
Peach High Juice Drink ROBINSONS	180.7	0.6	43.3	Tr	n/a
Pear Fruit Juice Concentrate MERIDIAN FOODS LTD	298	Tr	74.6	Tr	0
Pineapple 'C' LIBBY	44	0.1	10.9	Tr	Tr
Pineapple Fruit Juice DEL MONTE	52	0.4	12	Tr	n/a

All amounts per 100g/100ml unless otherwise stated	Cal kcal	Pro g	Carb g	Fat g	Fibre g
Pineapple Juice					
unsweetened	**41**	0.3	10.5	0.1	n/a
BRITVIC	**50.6**	0.4	11.1	0.1	n/a
Pink Grapefruit High Juice Drink ROBINSONS	**189.2**	0.2	45.3	Tr	n/a
Pink Grapefruit Juice with Bits					
DEL MONTE	**41**	0.5	9.1	Tr	n/a
Raspberry & Lemon Fruit Spring Drink ROBINSONS	**39.1**	Tr	9.3	Tr	n/a
Raspberry & Lovage Cordial					
BOTTLE GREEN	**27.3**	Tr	6.8	Tr	0
Ribena Berry Burst Juice Drink					
GLAXO SMITHKLINE	**40**	Tr	9.9	0	0
really light	**3**	Tr	0.6	0	0
Ribena Blackcurrant Juice Drink					
GLAXO SMITHKLINE	**45**	Tr	10.9	0	0
ready to drink	**51**	Tr	12.6	0	0
really light	**3**	Tr	0.5	0	0
Spiced Berry Cordial BOTTLE GREEN	**33**	0	8.2	0	0
Summer Fruits Squash ROBINSONS	**56**	0.1	12.8	Tr	n/a
Summer Fruits, High Juice					
ROBINSONS	**202.6**	0.2	49.3	Tr	n/a
no added sugar	**9.6**	0.1	1.2	Tr	n/a

All amounts per 100g/100ml unless otherwise stated	Cal kcal	Pro g	Carb g	Fat g	Fibre g
Tomato Juice	**14**	0.8	3	Tr	n/a
DEL MONTE	**19**	0.8	3.5	Tr	n/a
NAPOLINA	**16**	0.7	3.4	Tr	n/a
Cocktail BRITVIC	**20.7**	0.9	3.6	0.1	n/a
Tropical Fruit Burst DEL MONTE	**45**	0.2	10.9	Tr	n/a
Tropical Fruit Juice DEL MONTE	**50**	0.5	11	Tr	n/a
Watermelon World Fruits Juice Drink DEL MONTE	**46**	0.1	11	Tr	n/a
Water, flavoured, all flavours	**1**	Tr	Tr	0	0

See also: **KID'S FOODS**

FIZZY DRINKS

	Cal kcal	Pro g	Carb g	Fat g	Fibre g
7 Up PEPSI					
original	**46**	0	11.4	0	0
diet	**1.1**	0	n/a	0	n/a
Apple & Elderflower Pressé					
BOTTLE GREEN	**26**	Tr	6.4	Tr	0
Apple Soft Drink TANGO	**28.7**	Tr	6.8	Tr	n/a
low calorie	**4.5**	Tr	0.8	Tr	n/a
Bitter Lemon					
BRITVIC	**35.5**	Tr	8.3	Tr	n/a
SCHWEPPES	**33.9**	Tr	8.2	0	n/a
low calorie BRITVIC	**3.3**	Tr	0.2	Tr	n/a

All amounts per 100g/100ml unless otherwise stated	Cal kcal	Pro g	Carb g	Fat g	Fibre g
Slimline SCHWEPPES	**2.1**	Tr	0	0	n/a
Blackcurrant Pressé BOTTLE GREEN	**30**	0	7.4	0	0
Blueberry Pressé BOTTLE GREEN	**30**	0	7.4	0	0
Canada Dry Ginger Ale					
SCHWEPPES	**37.5**	Tr	9.1	0	n/a
Cherry Coke COCA-COLA	**45**	0	11	0	n/a
Cherry Soft Drink TANGO	**28.5**	Tr	6.8	Tr	n/a
Citrus Pressé BOTTLE GREEN	**24**	0	6.1	0	0
Coca-Cola COCA-COLA					
original	**43**	0	10.6	0	n/a
caffeine-free, diet	**0.4**	0	0	0	n/a
diet	**0.4**	0	0	0	n/a
with lemon, diet	**1.4**	0	0	0	n/a
vanilla	**43**	0	10.7	0	n/a
vanilla, diet	**0.4**	0	0.1	0	n/a
Cranberry Pressé BOTTLE GREEN	**30**	0	7.4	0	0
Cream Soda IDRIS	**21.4**	0	5.3	0	n/a
Dandelion & Burdock					
BARR	**19.6**	Tr	4.9	Tr	n/a
IDRIS	**22.1**	0	5.4	Tr	n/a
diet BARR	**1**	Tr	0.2	Tr	n/a
Elderflower Pressé BOTTLE GREEN	**35**	0	8.9	0	0
light	**12.8**	0	3.1	0	0

All amounts per 100g/100ml unless otherwise stated	Cal kcal	Pro g	Carb g	Fat g	Fibre g
Fanta COCA-COLA					
icy lemon	**50**	0	12	0	n/a
icy lemon, light	**2**	0	0.4	0	n/a
orange	**43**	0	10.5	0	n/a
orange, light	**3**	0	0.5	0	n/a
Fruit Fling Soft Drink TANGO	**30.6**	Tr	7.3	Tr	n/a
Ginger Ale, American BRITVIC	**37.6**	0	9.2	0	n/a
Ginger Ale, Dry SCHWEPPES	**15.9**	0	3.8	0	n/a
Ginger Beer IDRIS	**35.1**	Tr	8.5	0	n/a
Ginger Pressé BOTTLE GREEN	**28**	0	6.8	0	0
Irn Bru BARR	**41**	Tr	10.1	Tr	0
diet	**0.7**	Tr	Tr	Tr	0
Lemonade, bottled	**22**	Tr	5.8	0	n/a
CORONA	**10.6**	Tr	2.3	0	n/a
R WHITES	**22.6**	0	5.4	Tr	n/a
Lemonade, Premium R WHITES	**26.1**	Tr	6.2	Tr	n/a
low calorie R WHITES	**1.6**	Tr	Tr	Tr	n/a
Limeflower Pressé BOTTLE GREEN	**22**	0	5.4	0	0
Lucozade Glucose Drink GLAXO SMITHKLINE					
forest fruits	**70**	Tr	17.1	0	n/a
lemon	**70**	Tr	16.9	0	n/a
lemon lime	**70**	Tr	17	0	n/a

All amounts per 100g/100ml unless otherwise stated	Cal kcal	Pro g	Carb g	Fat g	Fibre g
orange	**70**	Tr	17.2	0	n/a
original	**73**	Tr	17.9	0	n/a
tropical	**70**	Tr	17.2	0	n/a
Lucozade Isotonic Drink					
GLAXO SMITHKLINE					
all flavours, sparkling	**28**	Tr	6.4	0	n/a
all flavours, still	**28**	Tr	.6.4	0	n/a
Oasis COCA-COLA					
Citrus Punch	**43.1**	n/a	10.4	n/a	n/a
Summer Fruits	**41.7**	n/a	10.1	n/a	n/a
Summer Fruits, light	**5**	n/a	0.9	n/a	n/a
Orange Soft Drink					
TANGO	**29.2**	Tr	6.7	Tr	n/a
low calorie TANGO	**5.4**	Tr	0.7	Tr	n/a
Orangina BARR	**41.2**	Tr	10.2	Tr	n/a
diet	**6**	0.1	1.2	0	n/a
Pepsi PEPSI	**44**	0	11.1	0	n/a
Diet	**0.3**	0.1	0.1	0	n/a
Tizer BARR	**26.3**	Tr	6.5	Tr	n/a
Tonic Water BRITVIC	**26.1**	0	6.2	0	n/a
SCHWEPPES	**21.8**	0	5.1	0	n/a
low calorie BRITVIC	**1.4**	Tr	0	0	n/a
Slimline SCHWEPPES	**1.8**	0	0	0	n/a
Water, flavoured, all flavours	**1**	Tr	Tr	0	0

All amounts per 100g/100ml unless otherwise stated	Cal kcal	Pro g	Carb g	Fat g	Fibre g
COFFEE & TEA					
Alta Rica NESCAFÉ	**98**	13.8	10	0.3	21
Blend 37 NESCAFÉ	**97**	14	10	0.1	20.4
Cappuccino NESCAFÉ					
café caramel	**423**	9.2	64.6	14.1	0
café hazelnut	**428**	9.3	66	14.1	0
café vanilla	**430**	9.3	64.6	14.9	0
decaffeinated	**428**	11.6	62.6	14.6	0
double choca mocha	**408**	9.2	68	11	0
latte	**507**	14.2	43.7	30.6	0
mocha	**418**	8.5	66.6	13.1	0
original	**444**	11.7	60.3	17.4	0
unsweetened	**464**	15	47.3	23.8	0
Coffee					
infusion, 5 minutes, average	**2**	0.2	0.3	Tr	n/a
instant, powdered	**75**	14.6	4.5	Tr	n/a
Coffeemate NESCAFÉ					
per 6.5g tsp	**26**	0.2	3.7	2.2	0
virtually fat free	**20**	0.1	4.2	0.3	0
Espresso, instant NESCAFÉ	**104**	15.2	10	0.4	11.5
Gold Blend NESCAFÉ	**102**	14.4	10	0.5	7.3
decaffinated	**101**	14.9	10	0.2	8.4
half caffeinated	**106**	15.9	10	0.3	11.7
Ice Tea LIPTON'S					
lemon	**28**	0	6.7	0	n/a

All amounts per 100g/100ml unless otherwise stated	Cal kcal	Pro g	Carb g	Fat g	Fibre g
mango	**33**	0	8.1	0	n/a
peach	**29**	0	6.9	0	n/a
peach lite	**1**	0	0	0	n/a
Lyle's Coffee Syrup TATE & LYLE					
almond	**245**	Tr	61	Tr	0
caramel	**329**	Tr	83	Tr	0
chocolate	**275**	Tr	69	Tr	0
cinnamon	**279**	Tr	69	Tr	0
hazelnut	**329**	Tr	83	Tr	0
Irish cream	**329**	Tr	83	Tr	0
vanilla	**329**	Tr	83	Tr	0
Nescafé Original NESCAFÉ	**103**	15.4	10	0.2	13.4
decaffeinated	**101**	14.9	10	0.2	8.4
half caffeinated	**106**	15.9	10	0.3	11.7
Tea, infusion, black	**Tr**	0.1	Tr	Tr	n/a
Tea PG Tips	**Tr**	0	0	0	0
Scottish Blend	**Tr**	0	0	0	0

HOT/MILK DRINKS

Banana Nesquik, as sold NESTLÉ	**395**	0	97.3	0.5	0
fresh, each	**175**	8.1	26.7	3.9	0.7
Beef Concentrate Drink BOVRIL	**170**	21.7	20.5	0.1	0.1
Bournvita Powder	**375**	4.1	85.4	1.7	2.2
made with milk	**45**	0.5	10.2	0.2	0.3

All amounts per 100g/100ml unless otherwise stated	Cal kcal	Pro g	Carb g	Fat g	Fibre g
Chicken Concentrate Drink					
BOVRIL	**129**	9.7	19.5	1.4	2.1
Chocolate Nesquik, as sold	**377**	4.9	82.5	3	5
fresh, each NESTLÉ	**190**	8.8	28.8	4.3	1.3
Cocoa Powder	**312**	18.5	11.5	21.7	n/a
made with semi-skimmed milk	**57**	3.5	7	1.9	0.2
made with whole milk	**76**	3.4	6.8	4.2	0.2
organic GREEN & BLACK	**322**	23	10.5	21	0
Rowntree NESTLÉ	**310**	17.5	11.5	21.5	4.9
Drinking Chocolate, powder	**373**	5.4	79.7	5.8	N
made with semi-skimmed milk	**73**	3.6	10.9	2	Tr
made with whole milk	**90**	3.5	10.7	4	1
Galaxy Caramel Instant Hot Chocolate Drink MARS	**395**	7.4	71.3	9.9	n/a
made up with water	**111**	2.1	20	2.8	n/a
Galaxy Chocolate Drink MARS	**411**	7	68.7	12.1	n/a
Galaxy Hazelnut Instant Hot Chocolate Drink MARS	**394**	7.4	71	9.9	n/a
made up with water	**110**	2.1	19.9	2.8	n/a
Galaxy Instant Hot Chocolate Drink MARS	**411**	7	68.7	12.1	n/a
made up with water	**115**	2	19.2	3.4	n/a
Horlicks GLAXO SMITHKLINE made up with semi-skimmed milk	**184**	9.4	28.5	4.6	0.7

All amounts per 100g/100ml unless otherwise stated	Cal kcal	Pro g	Carb g	Fat g	Fibre g
made up with whole milk	230	9.2	28.3	9.1	0.7
Horlicks Light Chocolate Malt Drink GLAXO SMITHKLINE	382	8.3	74.7	7.7	3.1
Horlicks Light Hot Chocolate Drink GLAXO SMITHKLINE	403	8	74	8.3	2.7
Horlicks Light Instant Powder GLAXO SMITHKLINE	364	14.8	72.2	3.8	1.9
made up with water	116	4.7	23.1	1.2	0.6
Hot Chocolate, organic GREEN & BLACK	385	9.2	75.9	9	n/a
Options, as prepared OVALTINE					
Belgian chocolate	40	1.4	6	1.1	0.8
mint	40	1.3	6	1.1	0.8
orange	40	1.7	5.6	1.3	n/a
white chocolate	45	1.2	7	1.4	n/a
Ovaltine					
powder OVALTINE	360	7.3	78.3	1.9	2.5
made up with semi-skimmed milk	187	86.6	29.5	3.8	0.6
Ovaltine Chocolatey OVALTINE	358	9	67.1	5.9	2.8
made up with water	72	1.8	13.4	1.2	0.6
Strawberry Nesquik, as sold NESTLÉ	390	0	96.7	0.5	0
fresh, each	175	8.3	26	4	0.8

EGGS

All amounts per 100g/100ml unless otherwise stated	Cal kcal	Pro g	Carb g	Fat g	Fibre g
Eggs, chicken					
raw, whole	**151**	12.5	Tr	11.2	0
raw, white only	**36**	9	Tr	Tr	n/a
raw, yolk only	**339**	16.1	Tr	30.5	n/a
boiled	**147**	12.5	Tr	10.8	n/a
fried, in vegetable oil	**179**	13.6	Tr	13.9	n/a
poached	**147**	12.5	Tr	10.8	n/a
scrambled with milk, recipe	**257**	10.9	0.7	23.4	n/a
Eggs, duck, raw, whole	**163**	14.3	Tr	11.8	n/a
Omelette, recipe					
plain	**195**	10.9	0	16.8	n/a
cheese	**271**	15.9	Tr	23	n/a

FISH & SEAFOOD

All amounts per 100g/100ml unless otherwise stated	Cal kcal	Pro g	Carb g	Fat g	Fibre g
FISH & SEAFOOD					
Anchovies, canned in oil, drained	**191**	25.2	0	10	0
Cockles, boiled	**53**	12	Tr	0.6	n/a
Cod					
baked fillets	**96**	21.4	Tr	1.2	n/a
dried, salted, boiled	**138**	32.5	0	0.9	n/a
fillets YOUNG'S BLUECREST	**80**	18.3	Tr	0.7	Tr
in batter, fried	**247**	16.1	11.7	15.4	n/a
in crumbs, frozen, fried	**235**	12.4	15.2	14.3	n/a
in parsley sauce, frozen, boiled	**84**	12	2.8	2.8	n/a
poached fillets	**94**	20.9	Tr	1.1	n/a
steaks, grilled	**95**	20.8	Tr	1.3	n/a
Cod Roe, hard, fried	**202**	20.9	3	11.9	n/a
Coley Fillets, steamed	**105**	23.3	0	1.3	n/a
frozen YOUNG'S BLUECREST	**82**	18.3	Tr	1	0.1
Crab					
boiled	**128**	19.5	Tr	5.5	n/a
canned in brine, drained	**77**	18.1	Tr	0.5	n/a
Eels, jellied	**98**	8.4	Tr	7.1	n/a
Haddock					
frozen YOUNG'S BLUECREST	**81**	19	Tr	0.6	Tr
in crumbs, frozen, fried	**196**	14.7	12.6	10	n/a

All amounts per 100g/100ml unless otherwise stated	Cal kcal	Pro g	Carb g	Fat g	Fibre g
smoked, frozen YOUNG'S BLUECREST	85	20.2	Tr	0.5	0.1
smoked, steamed	101	23.3	0	0.9	n/a
steamed	89	20.9	0	0.6	n/a
Halibut, grilled	121	25.3	0	2.2	n/a
Herring					
raw	190	17.8	0	13.2	n/a
grilled	181	20.1	0	11.2	n/a
fried, flesh only	234	23.1	1.5	15.1	N
grilled, flesh only	199	20.4	0	13	0
Kippers					
raw	229	17.5	0	17.7	n/a
grilled	255	20.1	0	19.4	n/a
Lemon Sole					
steamed	91	20.6	0	0.9	n/a
goujons, baked	187	16	14.7	14.6	n/a
goujons, fried	374	15.5	14.3	28.7	n/a
Lobster, boiled	119	22.1	0	3.4	0
Mackerel					
raw	220	18.7	0	16.1	n/a
grilled	239	20.8	0	17.3	n/a
smoked	354	18.9	0	30.9	n/a
Mussels, boiled	87	17.2	Tr	2	0
Pilchards, canned in tomato sauce	126	18.8	0.7	5.4	Tr

All amounts per 100g/100ml unless otherwise stated	Cal kcal	Pro g	Carb g	Fat g	Fibre g
Plaice					
in batter, fried	**257**	15.2	12	16.8	0
in crumbs, fried	**228**	18	8.6	13.7	0
goujons, baked	**304**	8.8	27.7	18.3	N
goujons, fried	**426**	8.5	27	32.3	0
steamed	**93**	18.9	0	1.9	0
Prawns					
boiled	**99**	22.6	0	0.9	n/a
boiled, weighed in shells	**41**	8.6	0	0.7	0
boiled Lyons Seafoods	**61**	13.5	0	0.6	n/a
in shell Young's Bluecrest	**56**	13.9	0.1	0	0.1
king, Atlantic Young's Bluecrest	**68**	16.1	0.1	0.4	0.1
king, freshwater Lyons Seafoods	**70**	16.8	0	0.3	n/a
king, cooked & peeled	**96**	22	0	0.9	0
king, gourmet Lyons Seafoods	**51**	12	0	0.5	n/a
North Atlantic, peeled					
Young's Bluecrest	**99**	22.6	0	0.9	0
tiger king, cooked Lyons Seafoods	**61**	13.5	0	0.6	n/a
tiger, headless & unpeeled					
Lyons Seafoods	**84**	19.6	0	0.7	n/a
tiger, whole, raw	**77**	18	0	0.6	0
tropical Lyons Seafoods	**51**	12	0	0.5	n/a
tropical, cooked & peeled					
Lyons Seafoods	**53**	12	0	0.6	n/a
tropical, in brine Lyons Seafoods	**71**	14.3	2	0.7	n/a
Roe					
cod, hard, fried	**202**	20.9	3	11.9	n/a

All amounts per 100g/100ml unless otherwise stated	Cal kcal	Pro g	Carb g	Fat g	Fibre g
herring, soft, fried	**244**	21.1	4.7	15.8	N
Saithe: *see* **Coley**					
Salmon					
fillet, frozen YOUNG'S BLUECREST	**192**	19.6	0.1	12.6	5.7
fillet, wild pink, frozen					
YOUNG'S BLUECREST	**133**	21.5	0.5	5	Tr
grilled steak	**215**	24.2	0	13.1	n/a
in white wine sauce					
YOUNG'S BLUECREST	**159**	13.4	0.7	11.4	0.7
pink, canned, in brine, drained	**153**	23.5	0	6.6	n/a
smoked	**142**	25.4	0	4.5	n/a
steamed	**194**	21.8	0	11.9	n/a
Salt Cod: *see* **Cod**					
Sardines					
canned in oil, drained	**220**	23.3	0	14.1	n/a
canned in tomato sauce	**162**	17	1.4	9.9	n/a
Scampi Tails					
premium LYONS SEAFOODS	**230**	8.4	26	10.9	n/a
Wholetail YOUNG'S BLUECREST	**233**	12.1	20.3	11.5	0.9
Seafood Selection					
LYONS SEAFOODS	**81**	14.9	1.3	2.3	n/a
YOUNG'S BLUECREST	**88**	17.1	2.8	0.9	0
Shrimps					
canned, drained	**94**	20.8	Tr	1.2	n/a
frozen, without shells	**73**	16.5	Tr	0.8	n/a

All amounts per 100g/100ml unless otherwise stated	Cal kcal	Pro g	Carb g	Fat g	Fibre g
Skate					
battered, fried	**168**	14.7	4.9	10.1	n/a
fried in butter	**199**	17.9	4.9	12.1	0.2
skinned skate wings	**81**	19	0	0.5	0
Sole: *see* **Lemon Sole**					
Swordfish, grilled	**139**	22.9	0	5.2	n/a
Trout					
brown, steamed, flesh only	**135**	23.5	0	4.5	0
rainbow, grilled	**135**	21.5	0	5.4	n/a
Tuna, chunks/steaks, drained					
canned in brine	**99**	23.5	0	0.6	n/a
canned in oil	**189**	27.1	0	9	n/a
steak, frozen Young's Bluecrest	**170**	24.3	0.4	7.9	0
Whelks, boiled	**89**	19.5	Tr	1.2	n/a
Whitebait, in flour, fried	**525**	19.5	5.3	47.5	n/a
Whiting					
steamed, flesh only	**92**	20.9	0	0.9	n/a
in crumbs, fried	**191**	18.1	7	10.3	n/a
Winkles, boiled	**72**	15.4	Tr	1.2	n/a

BREADED, BATTERED OR IN SAUCES

Calamari, Battered					
Young's Bluecrest	**177**	7.8	13	10.4	1.5

All amounts per 100g/100ml unless otherwise stated	Cal kcal	Pro g	Carb g	Fat g	Fibre g
Cod Fillet Fish Fingers					
fried in oil	**238**	13.2	15.5	14.1	n/a
grilled	**200**	14.3	16.6	8.9	n/a
BIRDS EYE	**186**	13	15.6	7.9	0.7
Cod Fillets					
in natural crumb	**180**	11.1	17.9	7.4	0.8
Chip Shop YOUNG'S BLUECREST	**210**	11.5	14.3	12.1	0.6
Chip Shop, large					
YOUNG'S BLUECREST	**233**	11	15.1	14.6	0.6
in red pepper sauce BIRDS EYE	**65**	10	3.2	1.3	0.2
Cod Steak					
in batter, fried in oil	**247**	16.1	11.7	15.4	n/a
in crumbs, fried in oil	**235**	12.4	15.2	14.3	n/a
in Butter Sauce BIRDS EYE	**109**	9.8	5	5.5	0.1
in Butter Sauce, each					
YOUNG'S BLUECREST	**77**	11.3	2.1	2.6	0.5
in Crispy Batter BIRDS EYE	**228**	12.2	14.9	13.3	0.5
in Crunch Crumb BIRDS EYE	**220**	14.1	17.5	10.4	0.8
in Parsley Sauce BIRDS EYE	**90**	10.5	5.6	2.8	0.1
in Parsley Sauce, each					
YOUNG'S BLUECREST	**70**	10.1	2.5	2.2	0.6
Fish Bakes BIRDS EYE					
Italiano Bake	**101**	12	3.9	4.1	0.4
Vegetable Tuscany	**115**	13.1	4.3	5	0.2
Fish Cakes ROSS	**160**	7.4	15.9	7.4	1.2
Chip Shop YOUNG'S BLUECREST	**247**	7.1	20.5	15.1	1.4

All amounts per 100g/100ml unless otherwise stated	Cal kcal	Pro g	Carb g	Fat g	Fibre g
in Crunch Crumb, Cod BIRDS EYE	**186**	11.3	15.9	8.6	1
fried	**218**	8.6	16.8	13.4	n/a
Fish en Croute, each					
YOUNG'S BLUECREST	**474**	15.5	26.8	33.9	7.7
Fish Fingers					
100% fish fillet ROSS	**193**	10.7	17.7	8.8	0.8
Chip Shop YOUNG'S BLUECREST	**251**	9.3	16.6	16.4	1.2
fried in oil	**233**	13.5	17.2	12.7	0.6
grilled	**214**	15.1	19.3	9	0.7
Crispy Batter BIRDS EYE	**236**	10.5	17	14	0.5
grilled BIRDS EYE	**187**	12.7	16.7	7.7	0.7
Fish Portions					
battered ROSS	**203**	10.4	16.1	10.8	0.8
garlic & herbs YOUNG'S BLUECREST	**222**	11	16.2	12.6	1.4
in butter sauce BIRDS EYE	**100**	13	2.6	4.3	0.1
in Crispy Batter BIRDS EYE	**198**	12.6	14.2	10.1	0.6
in Seasoned Breadcrumb BIRDS EYE	**179**	12.7	15	7.6	0.6
lemon & pepper YOUNG'S BLUECREST	**218**	10.3	15.3	12.9	4.3
Fish Steaks in Butter Sauce ROSS	**84**	9.1	3.2	3.9	0.1
Fish Steaks in Parsley Sauce ROSS	**82**	9.1	3.1	3.7	0.1
Fish Steaks, Chip Shop YOUNG'S BLUECREST	**240**	10.2	15.1	15.4	0.9

All amounts per 100g/100ml unless otherwise stated	Cal kcal	Pro g	Carb g	Fat g	Fibre g
Haddock, in crumbs, fried in oil	**196**	14.7	12.6	10	n/a
in crumbs BIRDS EYE	**199**	14.3	14.9	9.1	0.6
Haddock Fillet Fish Fingers					
BIRDS EYE	**185**	12.5	15.6	8.1	0.7
Haddock Fillets					
Chip Shop, large					
YOUNG'S BLUECREST	**222**	11.7	14.3	13.3	0.6
in Beer Batter BIRDS EYE	**204**	14.3	13.6	10.3	0.5
in Cheese Sauce BIRDS EYE	**88**	11	2.6	3.8	0.1
in Leek & Cheese Sauce BIRDS EYE	**87**	11	2.4	3.7	0.2
Haddock Mornay YOUNG'S BLUECREST	**122**	12.6	2	7.1	0.3
Haddock Steaks					
in Crispy Batter BIRDS EYE	**228**	12.5	14.9	13.2	0.5
in Crunch Crumb BIRDS EYE	**220**	14.1	17.5	10.4	0.8
Hoki, New Zealand					
YOUNG'S BLUECREST	**176**	14.3	11.7	8.7	0.8
Lemon Sole Goujons					
YOUNG'S BLUECREST	**226**	12.2	20.3	10.6	1.1
Mussels in a creamy garlic butter sauce YOUNG'S BLUECREST	**88**	9	5.2	3.5	0.6
Plaice					
Florentine YOUNG'S BLUECREST	**136**	10.6	2.6	9.3	1.6
in batter, fried in oil	**257**	15.2	12	16.8	n/a
in crumbs, fried, fillets	**228**	18	8.6	13.7	n/a

All amounts per 100g/100ml unless otherwise stated	Cal kcal	Pro g	Carb g	Fat g	Fibre g
Prawn Cocktail LYONS SEAFOODS	**429**	5.7	4.5	42.9	n/a
lite YOUNG'S BLUECREST	**109**	10.4	3.8	5.8	0
Prawns					
Hot & Spicy Crispy					
YOUNG'S BLUECREST	**230**	8.9	22.7	11.5	0.9
Hot 'n' Spicy LYONS SEAFOODS	**275**	6.5	32.1	14.3	n/a
Prawns, Popcorn LYONS SEAFOODS	**280**	9.1	18.9	19.4	n/a
Salmon Bites YOUNG'S BLUECREST	**223**	16.2	14.1	11.3	1.1
Salmon Grills YOUNG'S BLUECREST	**173**	19.3	5.7	8.1	0
Salmon Fillets in Dill Sauce					
BIRDS EYE	**106**	13	2.7	4.8	0
wild, in dill sauce BIRDS EYE	**93**	12	2.8	3.8	0.1
Scamp Bites ROSS	**202**	9.4	21.2	8.8	1
Scampi in Breadcrumbs					
frozen, fried	**237**	9.4	20.5	13.6	n/a
Scampi, whole in batter					
YOUNG'S BLUECREST	**212**	9.8	17.1	11	1.7
Seafood Cocktail LYONS SEAFOODS	**72**	14	2	1.8	n/a
Seafood Sticks YOUNG'S BLUECREST	**95**	8.1	14.5	0.4	1
Squat Lobster Wholetails					
YOUNG'S BLUECREST	**197**	9.8	20.1	8.6	1.1
Tuna Grills YOUNG'S BLUECREST	**214**	20.2	6	12.1	0
Whiting, in crumbs, fried	**191**	18.1	7	10.3	n/a

All amounts per 100g/100ml unless otherwise stated	Cal kcal	Pro g	Carb g	Fat g	Fibre g
MEALS					
Admiral's Pie YOUNG'S BLUECREST	105	4.8	10.9	4.6	0.7
Fish & Prawn Crumble, each YOUNG'S BLUECREST	474	21.6	36.3	27	4.7
Mature Cheddar Fish Bake, each YOUNG'S BLUECREST	171	20.3	7	6.8	1
Fish & Prawn Crumble YOUNG'S BLUECREST	127	5.8	9.7	7.2	1.3
Fish & Smoked Cheese with Sauté Potatoes YOUNG'S BLUECREST	151	6.2	12.5	8.5	1.1
Fish Pie, recipe	102	8	12.3	3	0.7
Fisherman's Pie YOUNG'S BLUECREST	113	7.1	8.4	5.6	1.5
Kedgeree, recipe	176	16	8	9.1	n/a
Mariner's Pie YOUNG'S BLUECREST	128	5	13.9	5.9	1
Mediterranean Fish Bake, each YOUNG'S BLUECREST	144	18.1	7.6	4.7	1.7
Ocean Crumble, low fat YOUNG'S BLUECREST	90	4.8	11.3	2.8	1.1
Ocean Pie WEIGHT WATCHERS	75	4.7	10.4	1.6	0.5
YOUNG'S BLUECREST	133	6.2	11.2	7	0.8
Prawn Kievs LYONS SEAFOODS	224	9.1	16	13.8	n/a

All amounts per 100g/100ml unless otherwise stated	Cal kcal	Pro g	Carb g	Fat g	Fibre g
Prawn Masala with Basmati Rice YOUNG'S BLUECREST	73	3.7	11.1	1.6	2
Salmon & Broccoli Wedge Melt WEIGHT WATCHERS	94	5.1	10.2	3.6	0.8
Salmon & Pasta YOUNG'S BLUECREST	137	7.8	16.6	4.4	1.2
Salmon & Prawns with Fusilli Pasta YOUNG'S BLUECREST	117	5.6	7	7.4	1.1
Salmon Crumble YOUNG'S BLUECREST	112	4.6	13	4.6	0.7
Salmon Mornay with Broccoli WEIGHT WATCHERS	91	9	9.1	2.1	0.7
Salmon Pie YOUNG'S BLUECREST	134	6.6	9.5	7.7	0.8
Scampi & Chips YOUNG'S BLUECREST	155	5.2	18.1	6.8	2
Seafood Paella YOUNG'S BLUECREST	127	4.7	19.7	3.3	0.1
Tuna Creamy Pasta Bake NAPOLINA	88	3.1	10.6	3.7	0.4
Tuna Twists Italiana WEIGHT WATCHERS	62	4.3	8.1	1.4	0.6

FLOUR & BAKING

All amounts per 100g/100ml unless otherwise stated	Cal kcal	Pro g	Carb g	Fat g	Fibre g
FLOUR					
Cornflour	**354**	0.6	92	0.7	n/a
BROWN & POLSON	**343**	0.6	83.6	0.7	0.1
Flour					
rye, whole	**335**	8.2	75.9	2	n/a
wheat, brown	**324**	12.6	68.5	2	n/a
wheat, white, breadmaking	**337**	11	70	1.4	3.1
wheat, white, plain	**336**	10	71	1.3	3.1
wheat, white, self-raising	**343**	11	72	1.2	2
wholemeal, plain	**308**	14	58	2.2	9
Ground Rice WHITWORTHS	**361**	6.5	86.8	1	0.5
PASTRY					
Pastry					
filo, uncooked	**311**	9	62	3	2
filo, sheets, uncooked JUS-ROL	**234**	8.1	52.1	2.7	2.1
flaky, cooked	**564**	5.6	46	41	n/a
puff, uncooked	**419**	5	30	31	1.6
puff, uncooked JUS-ROL	**401**	5.6	31.2	28.6	1.4
shortcrust, cooked	**524**	6.6	54.3	32.6	n/a
shortcrust, block, uncooked JUS-ROL	**462**	7	38.7	31	1.7
shortcrust, mix WHITWORTHS	**467**	7.4	60.8	23.2	2.3
wholemeal, cooked	**501**	8.9	44.6	33.2	n/a
vol-au-vent cases JUS-ROL	**401**	5.6	31.2	28.6	1.4

All amounts per 100g/100ml unless otherwise stated	Cal kcal	Pro g	Carb g	Fat g	Fibre g
BAKING AGENTS					
Baking Powder	**163**	5.2	37.8	0	n/a
Yeast, bakers					
compressed	**53**	11.4	1.1	0.4	n/a
dried	**169**	35.6	3.5	1.5	n/a
MIXES					
Batter Mix, Quick WHITWORTHS	**338**	9.3	77.2	1.2	3.7
Carmelle Mix GREEN'S	**83**	2.8	15	1.3	n/a
Cheesecake Mix GREEN'S	**278**	5.1	38.1	11.7	0.6
Crumble Mix WHITWORTHS	**422**	5.5	67.6	16.3	1.5
Egg Custard Mix, no bake GREEN'S	**96**	4.4	14.1	2.4	0.5
Lemon Meringue Crunch Mix GREEN'S	**249**	2.5	39	9	n/a
Lemon Pie Filling Mix, Royal GREEN'S	**110**	0.7	23.4	1.5	n/a
Madeira Loaf Mix GREEN'S	**339**	4.9	56	12.4	n/a
Mississippi Mud Pie GREEN'S	**323**	4	37.5	17.5	n/a
Pancake Mix WHITWORTHS	**322**	13.4	65.9	2.5	2.3
Strawberry Cheesecake GREEN'S	**258**	3	31.5	12	n/a

All amounts per 100g/100ml unless otherwise stated	Cal kcal	Pro g	Carb g	Fat g	Fibre g
Toffee Cheesecake GREEN'S	**342**	3.2	37.5	19.3	n/a
Victoria Sponge Mix GREEN'S	**367**	6	52	15	n/a

SUNDRIES

Cherries					
cocktail BURGESS	**247**	0.3	61.4	0	10
glacé	**251**	0.4	66.4	Tr	n/a
Cherry Pie Filling	**82**	0.4	21.5	Tr	n/a
Ginger, glacé WHITWORTHS	**304**	0.2	74.2	0.7	n/a
Lemon Juice, fresh	**7**	0.3	1.6	Tr	n/a
bottle JIF	**24**	0.5	2	Tr	0.1
Lime Juice, bottled JIF	**27**	0.5	0.7	Tr	n/a
Marzipan					
homemade	**462**	10.4	50.1	25.8	N
retail	**389**	5.3	67.6	12.7	N
Mincemeat	**274**	0.6	62.1	4.3	n/a
CHIVERS	**282**	0.6	63.6	2.8	n/a
with Courvoisier CHIVERS	**292**	1.5	60.7	4.8	n/a
Mixed Peel	**231**	0.3	59.1	0.9	n/a
Royal Icing TATE & LYLE	**390**	1.4	97.5	0	0

FRUIT & VEGETABLES

All amounts per 100g/100ml unless otherwise stated	Cal kcal	Pro g	Carb g	Fat g	Fibre g
FRUIT					
Apples, cooking					
flesh only	**35**	0.3	8.9	0.1	n/a
stewed with sugar	**74**	0.3	19.1	0.1	n/a
stewed without sugar	**33**	0.3	8.1	0.1	n/a
Apples, eating, flesh only	**45**	0.4	11.2	0.1	n/a
Apricots					
flesh & skin	**31**	0.9	7.2	0.1	n/a
canned in juice	**34**	0.5	8.4	0.1	n/a
canned in syrup	**63**	0.4	16.1	0.1	n/a
canned halves in syrup					
Del Monte	**78**	0.4	18.5	0.2	n/a
dried, ready to eat	**165**	3.9	36	0.6	6
Avocado Pears: *see* **Vegetables**					
Bananas					
peeled	**95**	1.2	23.2	0.3	n/a
dried, ready to eat					
Holland & Barrett	**221**	3.1	53.7	0.8	9.5
Blackberries	**25**	0.9	5.1	0.2	n/a
canned in fruit juice	**32**	0.6	7	0.2	1.8
John West	**33**	0.6	7.1	0.2	1.8
stewed with sugar	**56**	0.7	13.8	0.2	n/a
stewed without sugar	**21**	0.8	4.4	0.2	5.6

All amounts per 100g/100ml unless otherwise stated	Cal kcal	Pro g	Carb g	Fat g	Fibre g
Blackcurrants	**28**	0.9	6.6	Tr	n/a
canned in juice	**34**	0.6	8	Tr	n/a
canned in juice JOHN WEST	**33**	0.6	7.1	0.2	1.8
canned in syrup	**72**	0.7	18.4	Tr	3.6
stewed with sugar	**58**	0.7	15	Tr	n/a
Breadfruit, canned, drained	**66**	0.6	16.4	0.2	2.5
Cherries					
flesh & skin	**48**	0.9	11.5	0.1	n/a
canned in syrup	**71**	0.5	18.5	Tr	n/a
Cherries, black					
canned in juice PEK MORELLO	**87**	0.8	22.1	n/a	2
Cherries, cocktail: see BAKING					
Cherries, glacé: see BAKING					
Clementines					
flesh only	**37**	0.9	8.7	0.1	n/a
Coconut					
creamed	**669**	6	7	68.8	n/a
desiccated	**604**	5.6	6.4	62	n/a
Cranberries	**16**	0	4	0	4.2
Damsons					
flesh & skin	**38**	0.5	9.6	Tr	n/a
stewed with sugar	**74**	0.4	19.3	Tr	n/a

All amounts per 100g/100ml unless otherwise stated	Cal kcal	Pro g	Carb g	Fat g	Fibre g
Dates					
flesh & skin	124	1.5	31.3	0.1	n/a
block WHITWORTHS	288	3.3	68	0.2	n/a
chopped HOLLAND & BARRETT	253	2.8	64	0.2	4
stoned WHITWORTHS	287	3.2	68	0.2	3.9
Figs	122	0.4	7.2	Tr	6.9
dried, ready to eat	223	3.3	49	1.5	1.5
green, canned in syrup					
JOHN WEST	75	0.4	18	0.1	0.7
Fruit cocktail					
canned in juice	29	0.4	7.2	Tr	n/a
DEL MONTE	49	0.4	11.2	0.1	n/a
canned in syrup	57	0.4	14.8	Tr	n/a
DEL MONTE	75	0.4	18	0.1	n/a
Gooseberries	19	1.1	3	0.4	n/a
stewed with sugar	54	0.7	12.9	0.3	n/a
Grapefruit, flesh only	30	0.8	6.8	0.1	n/a
canned segments in juice					
DEL MONTE	49	0.6	10.9	0.1	n/a
Grapes, black/white, seedless	60	0.4	15.4	0.1	n/a
Greengages					
flesh & skin	34	0.5	8.6	Tr	1.6
stewed with sugar	107	1.3	26.9	0.1	1.5

All amounts per 100g/100ml unless otherwise stated	Cal kcal	Pro g	Carb g	Fat g	Fibre g
Guavas	**26**	0.8	5	0.5	n/a
canned in syrup	**60**	0.4	15.7	Tr	n/a
John West	**64**	0.4	15.7	Tr	3.1
Honeydew melon: see **Melon**					
Jackfruit	**88**	1.3	21.4	0.3	N
canned, drained	**104**	0.5	26.3	0.3	N
Kiwi fruit					
peeled	**49**	1.1	10.6	0.5	n/a
Lemons, whole	**19**	1	3.2	0.3	n/a
Lychees	**58**	0.9	14.3	0.1	n/a
canned in syrup	**68**	0.4	17.7	Tr	n/a
canned in syrup John West	**72**	0.4	17.7	Tr	0.6
Mandarin oranges					
canned in juice	**32**	0.7	7.7	Tr	n/a
Del Monte	**65**	0.6	10	0.1	n/a
canned in syrup	**52**	0.5	13.4	Tr	n/a
Del Monte	**61**	0.6	13.9	0.1	n/a
Mangos					
flesh only	**57**	0.7	14.1	0.2	n/a
canned in syrup	**57**	0.7	14.1	0.2	2.6
Melon, flesh only,					
cantaloupe-type	**19**	0.6	4.2	0.1	n/a
galia	**24**	0.5	5.6	0.1	n/a
honeydew	**28**	0.6	6.6	0.1	n/a
watermelon	**31**	0.5	7.1	0.3	n/a

All amounts per 100g/100ml unless otherwise stated	Cal kcal	Pro g	Carb g	Fat g	Fibre g
Nectarines, flesh & skin	**40**	1.4	9	0.1	n/a
Orange & Grapefruit Segments in Juice DEL MONTE	**48**	0.6	10.6	0	n/a
Oranges, flesh only	**37**	1.1	8.5	0.1	n/a
Papaya: *see* **Paw-paw**					
Passionfruit, flesh & pips only	**36**	2.6	5.8	0.4	n/a
Paw-paw					
flesh only	**36**	0.5	8.8	0.1	n/a
canned in juice	**65**	0.2	17	Tr	n/a
Peaches	**33**	1	7.6	0.1	n/a
canned in natural juice	**39**	0.6	9.7	Tr	n/a
DEL MONTE	**49**	0.5	11.2	0.1	n/a
canned in syrup	**55**	0.5	14	Tr	n/a
DEL MONTE	**77**	0.4	18.5	0.1	n/a
Pears	**40**	0.3	10	0.1	n/a
canned in natural juice	**33**	0.3	8.5	Tr	n/a
DEL MONTE	**45**	0.3	10.5	0.1	n/a
canned in syrup	**50**	0.2	13.2	Tr	n/a
DEL MONTE	**70**	0.2	17	0.1	n/a
Pineapple					
flesh only	**41**	0.4	10.1	0.2	n/a
canned in natural juice	**47**	0.3	12.2	Tr	n/a
DEL MONTE	**69**	0.4	15.5	0.1	n/a
canned in syrup	**64**	0.5	16.5	Tr	n/a

All amounts per 100g/100ml unless otherwise stated	Cal kcal	Pro g	Carb g	Fat g	Fibre g
DEL MONTE	75	0.4	17.5	0.1	n/a
canned in light syrup DEL MONTE	65	0.4	15	0.1	n/a
diced & dried HOLLAND & BARRETT	347	0.1	84.1	Tr	3.4
Plums	36	0.6	8.8	0.1	n/a
canned in syrup	59	0.3	15.5	Tr	n/a
Red JOHN WEST	73	0.3	18	Tr	0.8
Prunes					
canned in juice	79	0.7	19.7	0.2	n/a
canned in syrup	90	0.6	23	0.2	n/a
Prunes, dried: *see* **DRIED FRUIT & NUTS**					
Raisins: *see* **DRIED FRUIT & NUTS**					
Raspberries	25	1.4	4.6	0.3	n/a
stewed with sugar	48	0.9	11.5	0.1	1.2
canned in juice JOHN WEST	32	0.9	6.7	0.2	1.5
canned in syrup	88	0.6	22.5	0.1	n/a
canned in syrup JOHN WEST	82	0.8	19.3	0.2	1.5
frozen ROSS	26	1.2	4.7	0.3	4.4
Rhubarb	7	0.9	0.8	0.1	n/a
canned in syrup	31	0.9	7.6	Tr	n/a
stewed with sugar	48	0.9	11.5	0.1	n/a
stewed without sugar	7	0.9	0.7	0.1	1.3
Satsumas, flesh only	36	0.9	8.5	0.1	n/a
Strawberries	27	0.8	6	0.1	n/a
canned in syrup	65	0.5	16.9	Tr	n/a

All amounts per 100g/100ml unless otherwise stated	Cal kcal	Pro g	Carb g	Fat g	Fibre g
Summer Fruits, frozen Ross	**30**	0.9	6.3	0.1	3.4
Tangerines, flesh only	**35**	0.9	8	0.1	n/a
Watermelon, flesh only	**31**	0.5	7.1	0.3	n/a

See also: **DRIED FRUIT & NUTS**

VEGETABLES

	Cal kcal	Pro g	Carb g	Fat g	Fibre g
Artichoke, globe, base of leaves and heart, boiled	**18**	2.8	2.7	0.2	N
Artichoke, Jerusalem	**77**	2	17	0.1	1.6
flesh only, boiled	**41**	1.6	10.6	0.1	N
Asparagus					
soft tips only, boiled	**26**	3.4	1.4	0.8	n/a
canned, drained	**24**	3.4	1.5	0.5	2.9
Asparagus, Beans & Carrots Steam Bag, each Birds Eye	**30**	2	4.9	0.4	2.3
Aubergine, sliced, fried in corn oil	**302**	1.2	2.8	31.9	n/a
Avocado Pear	**190**	1.9	1.9	19.5	n/a
Bamboo Shoots sliced, canned	**7**	0.6	1	0.1	0.2
Beans, Broad					
canned	**82**	8	11	0.7	5
frozen, boiled	**81**	7.9	11.7	0.6	n/a
frozen, boiled Ross	**79**	7.9	10.7	0.6	6.5
prepack, shelled	**77**	6	12	0.6	0.6

All amounts per 100g/100ml unless otherwise stated	Cal kcal	Pro g	Carb g	Fat g	Fibre g
Beans, Green/French					
trimmed	**24**	1.9	3.2	0.5	n/a
trimmed, boiled	**22**	1.8	2.9	0.5	2.4
canned	**24**	1.5	3.8	0.3	2.6
frozen, whole	**25**	1.7	4.4	0.1	4.1
frozen, sliced	**27**	1.7	5	0	3.7
frozen, boiled	**25**	1.7	4.7	0.1	n/a
frozen, sliced, boiled Ross	**25**	1.8	4.4	0.1	4.1
Beans, Runner, trimmed, boiled	**18**	1.2	2.3	0.5	n/a

For dried & canned beans see: **BEANS, PULSES & CEREALS**

	Cal kcal	Pro g	Carb g	Fat g	Fibre g
Beansprouts, mung	**31**	2.9	4	0.5	n/a
stirfried in blended oil	**72**	1.9	2.5	6.1	n/a
Beetroot					
baby BAXTERS	**30**	1.5	6	Tr	1.2
baby HAYWARD'S	**27**	1.1	5.3	0.1	n/a
sliced HAYWARD'S	**25**	1.1	4.8	0.1	n/a
trimmed, peeled	**36**	1.7	7.6	0.1	n/a
trimmed, peeled, boiled	**46**	2.3	9.5	0.1	n/a
pickled, whole & sliced	**28**	1.2	5.6	0.2	n/a
pickled, all varieties BAXTERS	**109**	1	26	0.1	n/a
Broccoli florets, boiled	**24**	3.1	1.1	0.8	n/a
Premium Choice, frozen Ross	**24**	2.9	4.1	0.7	2.6
Brussels Sprouts					
trimmed, boiled	**35**	2.9	3.5	1.3	n/a
button, frozen, boiled Ross	**35**	3.5	2.4	1.3	4.3

All amounts per 100g/100ml unless otherwise stated	Cal kcal	Pro g	Carb g	Fat g	Fibre g
Cabbage (January King, Savoy, Summer)					
trimmed	**26**	1.7	4.1	0.4	n/a
boiled in unsalted water	**16**	1	2.2	0.4	n/a
white, trimmed	**27**	1.4	5	0.2	n/a
chopped, frozen Ross	**21**	1.3	3	0.5	2.9
Spring greens	**33**	3	3.1	1	n/a
Spring greens, boiled	**20**	1.9	1.6	0.7	n/a
Carrots					
old	**35**	0.6	7.9	0.3	n/a
old, boiled	**24**	0.6	4.9	0.4	n/a
young	**30**	0.7	6	0.5	n/a
young, boiled	**22**	0.6	4.4	0.4	n/a
canned	**20**	0.5	4.2	0.3	n/a
frozen, boiled	**22**	0.4	4.7	0.3	2.3
grated	**37**	0.6	8	0.3	2.4
Carrots, Broccoli & Sweetcorn, Steam Bag, each Birds Eye	**60**	3.1	10	1.1	2.6
Carrots, Cauliflower & Green Beans Steam Bag, each Birds Eye	**40**	2.4	6	0.6	2.6
Cassava					
baked	**155**	0.7	40.1	0.2	1.7
boiled	**130**	0.5	33.5	0.2	1.4
fresh	**142**	0.6	36.8	0.2	1.6
Cauliflower & Broccoli, frozen, boiled Ross	**25**	2.7	2.1	0.7	2.4

All amounts per 100g/100ml unless otherwise stated	Cal kcal	Pro g	Carb g	Fat g	Fibre g
Cauliflower	**34**	3.6	3	0.9	n/a
boiled	**28**	2.9	2.1	0.9	n/a
frozen, boiled Ross	**20**	2	1.9	0.5	1.2
Cauliflower, Peas & Carrots, each BIRDS EYE	**32**	2.2	4.8	0.4	2.6
Celeriac					
prepack	**29**	1.3	5	0.4	0.4
flesh only, boiled	**15**	0.9	1.9	0.5	3.2
Celery					
stem only	**7**	0.5	0.9	0.2	n/a
stem only, boiled	**8**	0.5	0.8	0.3	n/a
Chicory	**11**	0.5	2.8	0.6	n/a
Corn-on-the-cob					
boiled	**66**	2.5	11.6	1.4	n/a
mini corncobs, canned	**23**	2.9	2	0.4	n/a
mini corncobs, fresh/frozen, boiled	**24**	2.5	2.7	0.4	2
See also: **Sweetcorn**					
Courgettes (zucchini)					
trimmed	**18**	1.8	1.8	0.4	n/a
trimmed, boiled	**19**	2	2	0.4	n/a
trimmed, sliced, fried in corn oil	**63**	2.6	2.6	4.8	n/a
Cucumber, trimmed	**10**	0.7	1.5	0.1	n/a

Eggplant: *see* **Aubergine**

All amounts per 100g/100ml unless otherwise stated	Cal kcal	Pro g	Carb g	Fat g	Fibre g
Fennel, Florence	**12**	0.9	1.8	0.2	n/a
boiled	**11**	0.9	1.5	0.2	n/a
Garlic	**98**	7.9	16.3	0.6	n/a
purée	**423**	2.7	13	40	6
Gherkins, pickled	**14**	0.9	2.6	0.1	n/a
Ginger Root	**73**	1.7	15	0.7	2
Greens, spring: see **Cabbage**					
Gumbo: see **Okra**					
Kale, Curly	**33**	3.4	1.4	1.6	n/a
shredded & boiled	**24**	2.4	1	1.1	n/a
Kohlrabi	**23**	1.6	3.7	0.2	2.2
boiled	**18**	1.2	3.1	0.2	1.9
Lady's Fingers: see **Okra**					
Leeks					
trimmed	**22**	1.6	2.9	0.5	n/a
trimmed, chopped, boiled	**21**	1.2	2.6	0.7	n/a
Lettuce	**14**	0.8	1.7	0.5	n/a
iceberg	**13**	0.7	1.9	0.3	n/a
mediterranean salad	**19**	0.9	3.1	0.3	1.5
mixed leaf	**17**	1.1	2.9	0.1	2.7
Mange-tout	**32**	3.6	4.2	0.2	n/a
boiled	**26**	3.2	3.3	0.1	n/a
stir-fried	**71**	3.8	3.5	4.8	n/a

All amounts per 100g/100ml unless otherwise stated	Cal kcal	Pro g	Carb g	Fat g	Fibre g
Marrow					
flesh only	**12**	0.5	2.2	0.2	n/a
flesh only, boiled	**9**	0.4	1.6	0.2	n/a
Mixed Vegetables					
frozen, boiled Ross	**46**	3.1	7.1	0.7	3.6
Mooli: see **Radish, white**					
Mushrooms, common	**13**	1.8	0.4	0.5	n/a
boiled	**11**	1.8	0.4	0.3	1.1
canned	**12**	2.1	Tr	0.4	1.3
fried in oil	**157**	2.4	0.3	16.2	n/a
sliced, dried WHITWORTHS	**223**	16.5	40	1	22.9
Mushrooms, oyster	**8**	1.6	0	0.2	0.2
Mushrooms, shiitake					
cooked	**55**	1.6	12.3	0.2	N
dried	**296**	9.6	63.9	1	N
fresh	**8**	1.6	0	0.2	0.2
Mushrooms, straw					
canned, drained	**15**	2.1	1.2	0.2	N
Neeps (England): see **Swede**					
Neeps (Scotland): see **Turnip**					
Okra (gumbo, lady's fingers)	**31**	2.8	3	1	n/a
boiled	**28**	2.5	2.7	0.9	n/a
fresh	**41**	2	8	0.1	0.1
stir-fried	**269**	4.3	4.4	26.1	n/a

All amounts per 100g/100ml unless otherwise stated	Cal kcal	Pro g	Carb g	Fat g	Fibre g
Olives, pitted, in brine	**103**	0.9	Tr	11	n/a
Onions					
flesh only	**36**	1.2	7.9	0.2	n/a
boiled	**17**	0.6	3.7	0.1	0.7
cocktail/silverskin, drained	**15**	0.6	3.1	0.1	n/a
dried	**313**	10.2	68.6	1.7	12.1
fried in oil	**164**	2.3	14.1	11.2	n/a
pickled, drained	**24**	0.9	4.9	0.2	n/a
Parsnips, trimmed, peeled, boiled	**66**	1.6	12.9	1.2	n/a
frozen, boiled Ross	**65**	1.6	12	1.2	4.7
Peas					
no pod	**83**	6.9	11.3	1.5	n/a
boiled	**79**	6.7	10	1.6	n/a
canned	**80**	5.3	13.5	0.9	n/a
dried, boiled	**109**	6.9	19.9	0.8	5.5
frozen, boiled	**69**	6	9.7	0.9	n/a
Peas, Beans & Broccoli with Mint Steam Bag, each Birds Eye	**55**	3.8	4.2	2.5	3.7
Peas, Garden					
frozen Birds Eye	**62**	4.9	9	0.7	4.5
frozen, boiled Ross	**67**	5.9	8.9	0.9	5.1
Steam Bag, each Birds Eye	**50**	3.9	7.2	0.6	3.6
Peas, Mushy					
canned	**81**	5.8	13.8	0.7	n/a
Original Style, canned Batchelors	**77**	5.2	13.5	0.2	2.7

All amounts per 100g/100ml unless otherwise stated	Cal kcal	Pro g	Carb g	Fat g	Fibre g
Chip Shop Style, canned					
BATCHELORS	**78**	4.9	13.8	0.3	3.3
Chip Shop Mushy, frozen ROSS	**117**	7.5	23	0.2	1.8
Peas, Processed, canned	**99**	6.9	17.5	0.7	n/a
Bigga, canned BATCHELORS	**66**	5.6	10.1	0.3	4
Farrow's Giant, canned					
BATCHELORS	**77**	5.9	12.3	0.5	4.9
Small Processed BATCHELORS	**71**	5.4	11.1	0.6	5.1

See also: **Petit Pois**

See also: **BEANS, PULSES & CEREALS**

Peppers					
green, stalk & seeds removed	**15**	0.8	2.6	0.3	n/a
green, boiled	**18**	1	2.6	0.5	n/a
red, stalk & seeds removed	**32**	1	6.4	0.4	n/a
red, boiled	**34**	1.1	7	0.4	n/a
yellow, stalk & seeds removed	**26**	1.2	5.3	0.2	1.7
mixed, sliced, frozen	**28**	1.1	4.9	0.4	1.8
chilli, green	**20**	2.9	0.7	0.6	n/a
jalapeños, green DISCOVERY FOODS	**32**	n/a	3.4	0.7	n/a
jalapeños, sliced OLD EL PASO	**22**	1.3	3.4	0.3	n/a
Petits Pois	**100**	6.9	17.5	0.8	4.1
canned	**60**	4	11	0	5
frozen, boiled	**49**	5	5.5	0.9	n/a
frozen BIRDS EYE	**62**	5.4	8.7	0.6	3.8
frozen ROSS	**51**	4.2	10.4	1.2	4.6

All amounts per 100g/100ml unless otherwise stated	Cal kcal	Pro g	Carb g	Fat g	Fibre g
Petits Pois, Sugar Snap & Baby					
Corn Steam Bag, each BIRDS EYE	**45**	4.6	5.4	0.6	3.4
Potatoes, new					
boiled, peeled	**75**	1.5	17.8	0.3	n/a
boiled in skins	**66**	1.4	15.4	0.3	n/a
canned	**63**	1.5	15.1	0.1	n/a
Potatoes, old					
baked, flesh & skin	**136**	3.9	31.7	0.2	n/a
baked, flesh only	**77**	2.2	18	0.1	n/a
boiled, peeled	**72**	1.8	17	0.1	n/a
mashed with butter & milk	**104**	1.8	15.5	4.3	n/a
roast in oil/lard	**149**	2.9	25.9	4.5	n/a
Potato Powder, Instant					
made up with semi-skimmed milk	**70**	2.4	14.8	1.2	1
made up with skimmed milk	**66**	2.4	14.8	0.1	1
made up with water	**57**	1.5	13.5	0.1	n/a
made up with water SMASH	**60**	1.4	13.2	0.2	n/a
made up with whole milk	**76**	2.4	14.8	1.2	n/a

See also: **CHIPS, FRIES & SHAPED POTATO PRODUCTS**

Pumpkin					
flesh only	**13**	0.7	2.2	0.2	n/a
flesh only, boiled	**13**	0.6	2.1	0.3	n/a
Raddiccio	**14**	1.4	1.7	0.2	1.8
Radish, red	**12**	0.7	1.9	0.2	n/a

All amounts per 100g/100ml unless otherwise stated	Cal kcal	Pro g	Carb g	Fat g	Fibre g
Radish, white/mooli	15	0.8	2.9	0.1	N
Ratatouille, canned	50	1	7	2	1
Salad: *see also* **Lettuce**					
Salsify					
flesh only	27	1.3	10.2	0.3	3.2
flesh only, boiled	23	1.1	8.6	0.4	3.5
Shallots	20	1.5	3.3	0.2	n/a
Spinach	25	2.8	1.6	0.8	n/a
boiled	19	2.2	0.8	0.8	n/a
frozen, boiled	21	3.1	0.5	0.8	n/a
Spring Onions, bulbs & tops	23	2	3	0.5	n/a
Sprouts: *see* **Brussels Sprouts**					
Squash: *see* **Marrow**					
Sugar Snap, Leeks & Peas with Garlic Butter Steam Bag, each					
BIRDS EYE	90	4.4	5.8	5.5	3.6
Swede, flesh only, boiled	11	0.3	2.3	0.1	n/a
Sweet Potato, boiled	84	1.1	20.5	0.3	n/a
Sweetcorn, kernels					
canned, drained, re-heated	122	2.9	26.6	1.2	n/a
Niblets, canned GREEN GIANT	100	2.7	20.8	0.7	1.2
Niblets, no salt/sugar GREEN GIANT	77	2.6	16.7	0	2.6

All amounts per 100g/100ml unless otherwise stated	Cal kcal	Pro g	Carb g	Fat g	Fibre g
Niblets, Salad Crisp GREEN GIANT	70	2.7	13.3	0.7	2.7
Niblets with Peppers GREEN GIANT	82	2.6	17.9	0	1.3
on cob ROSS	65	2.5	10.6	1.4	1.3
Tomatoes	19	0.7	3.1	0.4	0.4
canned, whole	16	1	3	0.1	n/a
cherry	18	0.7	3.1	0.3	1
fried in oil	91	0.7	5	7.7	n/a
grilled	20	0.8	3.5	0.3	n/a
sun-dried	209	4.3	11	16.4	6.5
purée	76	5	14.2	0.3	n/a
passata	25	1.4	4.5	0.1	0.2
Tomatoes, chopped, canned					
NAPOLINA	22	1.1	3.5	0.4	n/a
for bolognese	24	1.4	5	Tr	n/a
with herbs	15	1.2	2.5	Tr	n/a
with onions & herbs	16	1.2	3	Tr	n/a
Turnip					
flesh only	23	0.9	4.7	0.3	n/a
flesh only, boiled	12	0.6	2	0.2	n/a
Water Chestnuts					
canned	28	1.7	4.7	0.3	2.6
canned AMOY	42	0.9	10.1	0	n/a
Wok vegetables FINDUS					
chinese	40	1.5	8	0.2	n/a
classic	30	2	5	0.3	n/a
Thai	35	1.5	7	0.3	n/a

All amounts per 100g/100ml unless otherwise stated	Cal kcal	Pro g	Carb g	Fat g	Fibre g
Yam					
flesh only	**114**	1.5	28.2	0.3	n/a
flesh only, boiled	**133**	1.7	33	0.3	n/a
Zucchini: *see* **Courgettes**					

JAMS, MARMALADES & SWEET SPREADS

All amounts per 100g/100ml unless otherwise stated	Cal kcal	Pro g	Carb g	Fat g	Fibre g
JAM, MARMALADE & HONEY					
Apricot Fruit Spread					
WEIGHT WATCHERS	110	0.3	27.2	0	0.5
organic MERIDIAN FOODS LTD	148	0.4	36	Tr	3
Apricot Jam					
Best HARTLEY'S	244	0.4	60.6	0	n/a
Family HARTLEY'S	256	0.3	63.7	0	n/a
reduced sugar HARTLEY'S	181	0.5	44.5	0	n/a
sucrose free DIETADE	260	0.3	64.4	Tr	n/a
Blackberry, Best HARTLEY'S	244	0.4	60.5	001	n/a
Black Cherry, Best HARTLEY'S	244	0.4	60.6	0	n/a
Blackcurrant Conserve,					
reduced sugar BAXTERS	193	0.3	48	0	1.3
Blackcurrant Fruit Spread					
WEIGHT WATCHERS	106	0.2	26.3	0	0.9
Carb Check HEINZ	54	0.5	12.8	0.1	2.7
organic MERIDIAN FOODS LTD	148	0.4	36	Tr	3
Blackcurrant Jam					
Best HARTLEY'S	244	0.4	60.6	0	n/a
Family HARTLEY'S	256	0.2	63.8	0	n/a
reduced sugar HARTLEY'S	180	0.5	44.5	0	n/a
sucrose free DIETADE	269	0.3	67	Tr	n/a

All amounts per 100g/100ml unless otherwise stated	Cal kcal	Pro g	Carb g	Fat g	Fibre g
Blueberry Fruit Spread, Wild					
organic MERIDIAN FOODS LTD	**148**	0.2	36	Tr	3.8
Blueberry Jam, Best HARTLEY'S	**244**	0.3	60.5	001	n/a
Cherries & Berries Fruit Spread,					
organic MERIDIAN FOODS LTD	**113**	0.5	27.1	0.3	0.8
Cranberry & Orange Fruit Spread,					
organic MERIDIAN FOODS LTD	**109**	0.5	26	0.3	1.1
Damson Jam, Best HARTLEY'S	**244**	0.2	60.8	0	n/a
Gooseberry Jam, Best HARTLEY'S	**245**	0.5	60.3	0.2	n/a
Grapefruit Fruit Spread					
MERIDIAN FOODS LTD	**138**	0.4	37.5	0.1	2.2
Honey					
comb	**281**	0.6	74.4	4.6	n/a
set	**306**	0.4	76	0	0
clear CHIVERS	**307**	0.4	76.4	Tr	0
clear GALES	**307**	0.4	76.4	Tr	n/a
Lemon Curd	**282**	0.6	62.7	4.9	N
GALES	**293**	0.7	61.4	4.9	n/a
Best HARTLEY'S	**288**	0.6	62.4	4	n/a
Marmalade	**261**	0.1	69.5	0	n/a
Breakfast HARTLEY'S	**260**	0.3	64.7	0	n/a
Fine Cut, Best HARTLEY'S	**260**	0.3	64.7	0	n/a
Lemon & Lime ROSE'S	**261**	0.2	64.7	0.1	n/a
Lemon ROSE'S	**252**	0.2	62.7	0.1	n/a

All amounts per 100g/100ml unless otherwise stated	Cal kcal	Pro g	Carb g	Fat g	Fibre g
Grapefruit ROSE'S	**252**	0.4	62.6	0	n/a
Lime ROSE'S	**265**	0.1	65.8	0.1	n/a
Olde English HARTLEY'S	**276**	0.3	68.7	0	n/a
Orange & Lemon ROSE'S	**264**	0.3	65.7	0.1	n/a
Orange ROSE'S	**252**	0.2	62.8	0	n/a
Orange, sucrose free DIETADE	**267**	0.2	66.4	Tr	n/a
Orange, reduced sugar HARTLEY'S	**180**	0.5	44.5	0	n/a
Orange, Lemon & Grapefruit, reduced sugar BAXTERS	**193**	0.2	48	Tr	0.2
Tangerine ROSE'S	**264**	0.1	65.9	0	n/a
Pink Grapefruit, reduced sugar HARTLEY'S	**180**	0.4	44.6	0	n/a
Shredless, Best	**260**	0.3	64.7	0	n/a
Thick Seville Orange, reduced sugar BAXTERS	**194**	0.3	48	Tr	0.3
Thin Seville Orange, reduced sugar BAXTERS	**194**	0.3	48	Tr	0.3
Morello Cherry Fruit Spread, organic MERIDIAN FOODS LTD	**148**	0.4	36	Tr	3
Pineapple & Ginger Fruit Spread MERIDIAN FOODS LTD	**137**	0.2	37.5	Tr	1.6
Pineapple Jam, Best HARTLEY'S	**244**	0.2	60.7	0.1	n/a
Raspberry Conserve reduced sugar BAXTERS	**197**	0.7	48	0.2	1.5

All amounts per 100g/100ml unless otherwise stated	Cal kcal	Pro g	Carb g	Fat g	Fibre g
Raspberry Fruit Spread					
WEIGHT WATCHERS	**111**	0.4	27.1	0.1	0.9
organic MERIDIAN FOODS LTD	**149**	0.5	36	Tr	2.6
Raspberry Jam					
Best HARTLEY'S	**244**	0.5	60.4	0	n/a
Family, seedless HARTLEY'S	**257**	0.5	63.4	0.1	n/a
reduced sugar HARTLEY'S	**181**	0.7	44.1	0.2	n/a
Seedless HARTLEY'S	**244**	0.5	60.4	0.1	n/a
sucrose free DIETADE	**259**	0.5	63.9	0.1	n/a
Red Cherry Jam, Best HARTLEY'S	**244**	0.4	60.6	0	n/a
Rhubarb & Ginger Jam reduced sugar BAXTERS	**194**	0.4	48	Tr	0.7
Seville Orange Fruit Spread					
WEIGHT WATCHERS	**111**	0.2	27.5	0	0.3
organic MERIDIAN FOODS LTD	**148**	0.4	36	Tr	2.2
Strawberry Conserve reduced sugar BAXTERS	**195**	0.4	48	0.1	0.7
Strawberry Fruit Spread					
WEIGHT WATCHERS	**115**	0.2	28.4	0	0.4
Carb Check HEINZ	**56**	0.3	13.6	Tr	0.5
organic MERIDIAN FOODS LTD	**147**	0.3	36	Tr	2.5
Strawberry Jam					
Best HARTLEY'S	**244**	0.4	60.6	0	n/a
Family HARTLEY'S	**256**	0.3	63.7	0	n/a
reduced sugar HARTLEY'S	**181**	0.4	44.5	0.1	n/a
sucrose free DIETADE	**257**	0.3	63.8	Tr	n/a

All amounts per 100g/100ml unless otherwise stated	Cal kcal	Pro g	Carb g	Fat g	Fibre g
NUT BUTTERS					
Almond Butter					
MERIDIAN FOODS LTD	**633**	25.5	6.5	56.1	7.4
Brazil Butter					
MERIDIAN FOODS LTD	**633**	16.8	3.5	52.8	3.4
Cashew Butter					
MERIDIAN FOODS LTD	**632**	24.3	17.4	51.7	3.2
Chocolate Nut Spread	**549**	6.2	60.5	33	n/a
Hazel Butter MERIDIAN FOODS LTD	**678**	16	5.4	65.9	6.3
Nutella FERRERO	**533**	6.5	57	31	n/a
Peanut Butter					
extra crunchy SUNPAT	**597**	21.9	12.6	51	n/a
crunchy	**606**	24	15	50	6
crunchy SUNPAT	**587**	23.6	10.3	50.1	n/a
organic MERIDIAN FOODS LTD	**606**	31	12.1	48.2	6.5
organic, no salt MERIDIAN FOODS LTD	**612**	31.2	12.2	48.7	6.5
smooth	**611**	23	15	51	6
smooth SUNPAT	**600**	27	14.5	48.2	n/a
super smooth SUNPAT	**599**	21	14.1	51	n/a
Tahini Paste	**607**	18.5	0.9	58.9	n/a
Walnut Butter MERIDIAN FOODS LTD	**649**	17.7	2	53.6	2.3

MEAT & POULTRY

All amounts per 100g/100ml unless otherwise stated	Cal kcal	Pro g	Carb g	Fat g	Fibre g
BACON & GAMMON					
Bacon, rashers, back					
dry fried	**295**	24.2	0	22	n/a
fat trimmed, grilled	**214**	25.7	0	12.3	n/a
grilled	**287**	23.2	0	21.6	n/a
microwaved	**307**	24.2	0	23.3	n/a
uncooked	**215**	16.5	0	16.5	n/a
uncooked, smoked WALL'S	**188**	16.2	0.5	13.5	n/a
uncooked, unsmoked WALL'S	**188**	16.2	0.5	13.5	n/a
Bacon, rashers, middle, grilled	**307**	24.8	0	23.1	n/a
Bacon, rashers, streaky					
fried	**335**	23.8	0	26.6	n/a
grilled	**337**	23.8	0	26.9	n/a
Gammon, joint, boiled	**204**	23.3	0	12.3	n/a
Gammon, rashers, grilled	**199**	27.5	0	9.9	n/a
SAUSAGES					
Beef sausages, grilled	**278**	13.3	13.1	19.5	0.7
Cumberland sausages, uncooked WALL'S	**314**	14.4	14.3	22.2	1.4
Frankfurters HERTA	**328**	12.5	2	30	Tr
Lincolnshire sausages, uncooked WALL'S	**307**	13	16	21.3	1.2

All amounts per 100g/100ml unless otherwise stated	Cal kcal	Pro g	Carb g	Fat g	Fibre g
Pork sausages					
fried	**308**	13.9	9.9	23.9	n/a
lean recipe, uncooked WALL'S	**132**	15.4	8.5	4.1	2.1
micro WALL'S	**330**	12.2	13.4	25.3	2.3
skinless, uncooked WALL'S	**313**	11.4	11.6	24.6	0.1
Pork & beef sausages, thick, uncooked WALL'S	**300**	9.3	18.5	21	1
Premium sausages, grilled	**292**	16.8	6.3	22.4	N
Saveloy	**296**	13.8	10.8	22.3	n/a
BEEF					
Beef, fore-rib, roasted	**300**	29.1	0	20.4	n/a
Beef, mince, stewed	**209**	21.8	0	13.5	0
Beef, rump steak					
lean, grilled	**177**	31	0	5.9	0
lean, fried	**183**	30.9	0	6.6	0
lean & fat, fried	**228**	28.4	0	12.7	n/a
Beef, silverside, lean only, boiled	**184**	30.4	0	6.9	n/a
Beef, stewing steak, lean & fat, stewed	**203**	29.2	0	9.6	n/a
Beef, topside					
lean only, roasted well-done	**202**	36.2	0	6.3	n/a
lean & fat, roasted	**244**	32.8	0	12.5	n/a

All amounts per 100g/100ml unless otherwise stated	Cal kcal	Pro g	Carb g	Fat g	Fibre g
Grillsteaks, grilled	**305**	22.1	0.5	23.9	n/a
Oxtail, stewed	**243**	30.5	0	13.4	n/a
Beef, sausages: *see* **SAUSAGES**					

LAMB

Lamb, breast					
lean only, roasted	**273**	26.7	0	18.5	n/a
lean & fat, roasted	**359**	22.4	0	29.9	n/a
Lamb, loin chops					
lean only, grilled	**213**	29.2	0	10.7	n/a
lean & fat, grilled	**305**	26.5	0	22.1	n/a
Lamb, cutlets					
lean only, grilled	**238**	28.5	0	13.8	n/a
lean & fat, grilled	**367**	24.5	0	29.9	n/a
Lamb, leg					
whole, lean only, roasted	**203**	29.7	0	9.4	n/a
whole, lean & fat, roasted	**240**	28.1	0	14.2	0
Lamb, mince, stewed	**208**	24.4	0	12.3	n/a
Lamb, stewing, lean only, stewed	**240**	26.6	0	14.8	n/a
Lamb, shoulder					
lean only, roasted	**218**	27.2	0	12.1	n/a
lean & fat, roasted	**298**	24.7	0	22.1	n/a

All amounts per 100g/100ml unless otherwise stated	Cal kcal	Pro g	Carb g	Fat g	Fibre g

PORK

Pork, belly rashers, lean & fat, grilled	**320**	27.4	0	23.4	n/a
Pork, loin chops, lean only, grilled	**184**	31.6	0	6.4	n/a
Pork, leg					
lean only, roasted	**182**	33	0	5.5	0
lean & fat, roasted	**215**	30.9	0	10.2	0
Pork, steaks, lean & fat, grilled	**198**	32.4	0	7.6	n/a
Pork, sausages: *see* SAUSAGES					

VEAL

Veal, escalope fried	**196**	33.7	0	6.8	0

CHICKEN

Chicken, breast					
in crumbs, fried	**242**	18	14.8	12.7	n/a
meat only, casseroled	**160**	28.4	0	5.2	n/a
meat only, grilled	**148**	32	0	2.2	n/a
meat only, stir fried	**161**	29.7	0	4.6	n/a
Chicken, drumsticks, meat & skin, roasted	**185**	25.8	0	9.1	n/a

All amounts per 100g/100ml unless otherwise stated	Cal kcal	Pro g	Carb g	Fat g	Fibre g
Chicken, leg quarter, meat & skin, roasted	**236**	20.9	0	16.9	n/a
Chicken, light & dark meat, roasted	**177**	27.3	0	7.5	n/a
Chicken, wing quarter, meat & skin, roasted	**226**	24.8	0	14.1	n/a
Chicken, light meat, roasted	**153**	30.2	0	3.6	n/a

TURKEY

Turkey, breast fillet, meat only, grilled	**155**	35	0	1.7	n/a
Turkey, dark meat, roasted	**177**	29.4	0	6.6	n/a
Turkey, light meat, roasted	**153**	33.7	0	2	n/a
Turkey, meat only, roasted	**166**	31.2	0	4.6	n/a

GAME

Duck					
meat only, roasted	**195**	25.3	0	10.4	n/a
meat, fat & skin, roasted	**423**	20	0	38.1	n/a
Duck, crispy, Chinese style	**331**	27.9	0.3	24.2	0
Goose, meat, fat & skin, roasted	**301**	27.5	0	21.2	n/a

All amounts per 100g/100ml unless otherwise stated	Cal kcal	Pro g	Carb g	Fat g	Fibre g
Pheasant, meat only, roasted	**220**	27.9	0	12	n/a
Rabbit, meat only, stewed	**114**	21.2	0	3.2	n/a
Venison, haunch, meat only, roasted	**165**	35.6	0	2.5	n/a

OFFAL

Black Pudding, dry fried	**297**	10.3	16.6	21.5	n/a
Heart, lamb, roasted	**226**	25.3	0	13.9	n/a
Kidney, lamb, fried	**188**	23.7	0	10.3	n/a
Kidney, ox, stewed	**138**	24.5	0	4.4	n/a
Kidney, pig, stewed	**153**	24.4	0	6.1	n/a
Liver, calf, fried	**176**	22.3	Tr	9.6	n/a
Liver, chicken, fried	**169**	22.1	Tr	8.9	n/a
Liver, lamb, fried	**237**	30.1	Tr	12.9	n/a
Liver, ox, stewed	**198**	24.8	3.6	9.5	n/a
Liver, pig, stewed	**189**	25.6	3.6	8.1	n/a
Tripe, dressed, raw	**33**	7.1	0	0.5	n/a
White Pudding	**450**	7	36.3	31.8	n/a

OILS & FATS

All amounts per 100g/100ml unless otherwise stated	Cal kcal	Pro g	Carb g	Fat g	Fibre g
OILS					
Crisp 'n' Dry SPRY	**828**	0	0	92	0
Coconut Oil	**899**	Tr	0	99.9	n/a
Corn Oil MAZOLA	**829**	0	0	92.1	0
Olive Oil	**899**	Tr	0	99.9	n/a
Delicato BERTOLLI	**820**	0	0	91	0
CARAPELLI	**822**	0	0	91.3	0
FILIPPO BERRIO	**822**	0	0	91.3	0
Extra Virgin BERTOLLI	**820**	0	0	91	0
FILIPPO BERRIO	**820**	0	0	91	0
NAPOLINA	**823**	0	0	91.6	0
OLIVIO	**828**	0	0	92	0
organic MERIDIAN FOODS LTD	**899**	Tr	0	99.9	0
Palm Oil	**899**	Tr	0	99.9	n/a
Peanut Oil	**899**	Tr	0	99.9	n/a
Rapeseed Oil	**899**	Tr	0	99.9	n/a
Safflower Oil	**899**	Tr	0	99.9	n/a
organic MERIDIAN FOODS LTD	**899**	Tr	0	99.9	0
Sesame Oil	**898**	0.2	0	99.7	n/a
roasted SHARWOOD	**826**	0.2	Tr	91.7	Tr
organic MERIDIAN FOODS LTD	**881**	Tr	0	99.9	0
organic, toasted MERIDIAN FOODS LTD	**881**	Tr	0	99.9	0

All amounts per 100g/100ml unless otherwise stated	Cal kcal	Pro g	Carb g	Fat g	Fibre g
Soya Oil	**899**	Tr	0	99.9	n/a
Sunflower Oil FLORA	**828**	0	0	92	0
organic MERIDIAN FOODS LTD	**899**	Tr	0	99.9	0
Sunflower Oil Seed	**899**	Tr	0	99.9	n/a
Vegetable Oil	**899**	Tr	0	99.9	0
Wheatgerm Oil	**899**	Tr	0	99.9	n/a
Wok Oil SHARWOOD	**811**	0.1	0.4	89.8	Tr

FATS

Cooking Fat					
COOKEEN	**900**	0	0	100	0
Crisp 'n' Dry, solid SPRY	**900**	0	0	100	0
White Flora FLORA	**900**	0	0	100	0
Dripping, beef	**891**	Tr	Tr	99	0
Ghee					
butter	**898**	Tr	Tr	99.8	n/a
palm	**897**	Tr	Tr	99.7	0
vegetable	**895**	Tr	Tr	99.4	n/a
Lard	**891**	Tr	0	99	n/a
Suet, shredded	**826**	Tr	12.1	86.7	n/a

PASTA

All amounts per 100g/100ml unless otherwise stated	Cal kcal	Pro g	Carb g	Fat g	Fibre g
Cooked Lasagne sheets BUITONI					
standard	**89**	3.1	18.1	0.4	n/a
verdi	**93**	3.2	18.3	0.4	n/a
Cooked Pasta, all shapes BUITONI					
standard	**89**	3.1	18.1	0.4	n/a
verdi	**93**	3.2	18.3	0.4	n/a
Dry Lasagne sheets BUITONI					
standard	**352**	11.2	72.6	1.9	n/a
verdi	**367**	12.8	75.2	1.7	n/a
Dry Pasta, all shapes					
Carb Check HEINZ	**292**	52.7	15.2	2.3	20.8
low carbohydrate CARB OPTION	**350**	28.5	34	1.5	21
standard BUITONI	**362**	12.2	74.4	1.7	n/a
verdi BUITONI	**367**	12.8	75.2	1.7	n/a
Fresh Egg Pasta					
conchiglie, penne, fusilli	**170**	7	31	2	1.4
Lasagne sheets	**150**	6	29	1.1	4.6
Spaghetti	**129**	5	24	1.4	1
Tagliatelle	**129**	5	24	1	1
Macaroni, boiled	**86**	3	18.5	0.5	n/a
Spaghetti					
cooked	**104**	3.6	22.2	0.7	n/a
wholemeal, cooked	**113**	4.7	23.2	0.9	N

All amounts per 100g/100ml unless otherwise stated	Cal kcal	Pro g	Carb g	Fat g	Fibre g
Stuffed Fresh Pasta					
meat ravioli	**211**	8	29	7	2.9
cheese ravioli	**256**	9	37	8	2.4
chicken & mushroom tortellini	**182**	6	26	6	2.4
garlic, basil & ricotta tortellini	**182**	6	26	6	2.6
ham & cheese tortellini	**170**	6	23	6	1.7
spinach & ricotta tortellini	**163**	6	24	4.8	2.7

CLASSIC PASTA SAUCES

See also: **COOKING SAUCES & MARINADES (ITALIAN)**

Amatriciana	**155**	4.4	5	13	1
Arrabbiata, fresh	**48**	1.2	7	1.7	0.7
Beef Bolognese Sauce, fresh	**77**	4.7	3.4	5	0.4
Bolognese Sauce, recipe, with meat	**161**	11.8	2.5	11.6	n/a
Carbonara					
fresh	**196**	6	4.8	17	0.5
fresh, low fat	**81**	5	5	4.5	0.5
Pesto					
creamy fresh	**45**	2.2	6	1.3	1.4
green LOYD GROSSMAN	**458**	4.3	11.9	43.7	n/a
jar	**374**	5	0.8	39	5
red LOYD GROSSMAN	**529**	5.4	10	51.9	n/a
red, jar	**358**	4.1	3.1	36.6	0.4

All amounts per 100g/100ml unless otherwise stated	Cal kcal	Pro g	Carb g	Fat g	Fibre g
rosso BERTOLLI	**389**	6.6	8.1	36.7	1.5
verdi BERTOLLI	**575**	5.7	4.3	59.5	3
Tomato & basil, fresh	**51**	1.8	8.8	0.9	1.3
Tomato Pasta Sauce, jar	**47**	2	6.9	1.5	n/a

TINNED PASTA

Bolognese Shells WEIGHT WATCHERS	**79**	3.4	13.4	1.4	0.4
Ravioli in Tomato Sauce HEINZ	**73**	3.1	13.2	0.8	0.3
Spaghetti Bolognese HEINZ	**79**	3.4	13.2	1.5	0.5
Spaghetti Hoops HEINZ	**53**	1.7	11.1	0.2	0.5
Spaghetti Hoops 'n' Hotdogs in a Smoky Bacon Sauce HEINZ	**76**	2.8	11	2.4	0.4
Spaghetti in Tomato Sauce					
CROSSE & BLACKWELL	**88**	3.3	15	1.7	n/a
HEINZ	**61**	1.7	13	0.2	0.5
no added sugar WEIGHT WATCHERS	**50**	1.8	10.1	0.2	0.6
Spaghetti with Sausages in Tomato Sauce HEINZ	**88**	3.5	10.8	3.4	0.5
Spicy Pepperoni Pasta HEINZ	**83**	2.9	9.1	3.9	0.5
Spicy Salsa Twists HEINZ	**75**	2.7	10.9	2.3	0.8

See also: **KIDS' FOOD**

PIZZA

All amounts per 100g/100ml unless otherwise stated	Cal kcal	Pro g	Carb g	Fat g	Fibre g
Americano SAN MARCO	**253**	10.3	28.9	10.7	1.8
Cheese & Onion Deep Topped					
Pizza, slices McVITIE'S	**223**	8.4	30.3	8.2	1.3
Cheese & Tomato Pizza					
recipe	**235**	9	24.8	11.8	1.5
deep pan base	**249**	12.4	35.1	7.5	n/a
deep pan ROSS	**270**	10.8	35.1	9.6	2.7
French bread base	**230**	10.6	31.4	7.8	N
thin base	**277**	14.4	33.9	10.3	n/a
fingers McCAIN	**230**	11.8	28.9	7.5	n/a
Chicken Provençal Pizza					
GOODFELLA'S	**272**	13.7	25.9	2.6	2.1
Familia, Thin & Crispy SAN MARCO					
Hawaiian	**231**	8.9	27.9	9.2	1.5
Margherita	**280**	10.5	28.1	13.9	1.5
Pepperoni	**287**	10.7	26.9	15.1	1.6
Four Cheese,					
deep dish, individual SAN MARCO	**271**	8.9	35.4	10.4	1.9
French Bread Pizza FINDUS					
Cheese & Tomato	**240**	11	31	7.5	1.5
Sticky BBQ	**230**	10	32	7	N/A
Ham & Pineapple, deep pan					
CHICAGO TOWN	**242**	11	30.3	8.5	1.5
deep dish, individual SAN MARCO	**238**	9.7	30.2	8.7	2

All amounts per 100g/100ml unless otherwise stated	Cal kcal	Pro g	Carb g	Fat g	Fibre g
deep pan, individual					
CHICAGO TOWN	**245**	9	31.8	9.1	1.5
Hawaiian Pizza					
GOODFELLA'S	**245**	10.9	27.9	9.9	2.1
deep pan ROSS	**244**	11.2	30.4	8.6	2.7
Hot & Spicy Deep Pan,					
individual CHICAGO TOWN	**252**	9.3	30.5	10.3	1.5
Margherita Pizza					
GOODFELLA'S	**280**	12.7	29	12.5	2.2
Micro Pizza MCCAIN					
cheese & tomato	**308**	13.7	26	16.6	n/a
pepperoni	**324**	12.2	28.6	17.9	n/a
spicy chicken	**287**	12.1	27.7	14.2	n/a
Napola SAN MARCO	**223**	11.1	31.1	6	2.1
Pepperoni Pizza					
GOODFELLA'S	**303**	11.6	28.1	16	2.2
deep dish, individual SAN MARCO	**291**	11.1	31.1	13.6	1.7
deep pan CHICAGO TOWN	**263**	10.6	29.2	11.5	1.7
deep pan ROSS	**267**	10.9	35.3	9.1	2.2
deep pan, individual CHICAGO TOWN	**307**	10.9	29.9	16	1.9
Pizza Bases NAPOLINA					
deep pan	**298**	8.5	56	4.4	n/a
mini	**298**	8.5	56	4.4	n/a

All amounts per 100g/100ml unless otherwise stated	Cal kcal	Pro g	Carb g	Fat g	Fibre g
standard	**298**	8.5	56	4.4	n/a
stone baked	**274**	8.5	55	2.2	n/a
Pizza Topping NAPOLINA					
spicy tomato	**66**	1.6	9	2.6	1
tomato, cheese, onion & herbs	**80**	3	8.1	4	0.9
tomato, herbs & spices	**67**	1.5	9.4	2.6	0.8
Pizzeria SAN MARCO					
Mozzarella	**240**	10.9	30.6	9.3	3.4
Supreme	**248**	10.9	30.6	9.3	3.4
Snack Attack SAN MARCO					
chicken & onion	**269**	12.5	30.1	10.9	1.7
Triple Cheese Extra Thin Crust CHICAGO TOWN	**286**	11.9	28.2	13.9	1.5

See also: **FAST FOOD**

QUICHES, PIES & SAVOURY PASTRIES

All amounts per 100g/100ml unless otherwise stated	Cal kcal	Pro g	Carb g	Fat g	Fibre g
Beef & Beer Pie, canned PRINCE'S	179	10.2	16.1	8.2	n/a
Beef & Kidney Pie, canned TYNE BRAND	154	8.7	13.3	8.1	n/a
Beef & Mushroom Pie, canned TYNE BRAND	162	10.1	11.8	8.3	n/a
Beef & Potato Pie, canned TYNE BRAND	191	7.1	22.2	8.2	n/a
Beef & Vegetable Pie, canned TYNE BRAND	185	6.5	22.5	7.7	n/a
Chicken & Asparagus Pie, frozen McDOUGALL'S	288	8	19	20	0.9
Chicken & Mushroom Pie, canned FRAY BENTOS	162	6.7	11.6	9.9	n/a
canned PRINCE'S	194	9.9	18	9.1	n/a
individual	321	8	25	21	1
Cheese & Onion Pie, individual	325	7	27	21	1.1
Chicken & Vegetable Pie, canned TYNE BRAND	162	4.7	14.3	9.6	n/a
Chicken, Ham & Mushroom Pie, frozen McDOUGALL'S	261	9	18	17	0.8
Chicken Lattice BIRDS EYE Bacon & Cheese, each	390	18	28	23	2

All amounts per 100g/100ml unless otherwise stated	Cal kcal	Pro g	Carb g	Fat g	Fibre g
Cheese & Broccoli, each	**385**	17	30	22	1.5
Tomato & Basil, each	**340**	18	25	19	2.7
Chicken Pie, frozen, each					
BIRDS EYE	**460**	13	35	30	2.1
Cornish Pastie	**267**	6.7	25	16.3	n/a
giant ROSS	**228**	6.5	24.5	12	1
Game Pie	**381**	12.2	34.7	22.5	n/a
Minced Beef & Onion Deep Pie,					
frozen ROSS	**249**	6	24.6	14.5	1
Minced Beef & Onion Pastie,					
giant, frozen ROSS	**259**	6	28	14.2	1.2
Minced Beef & Onion Pie	**241**	7	24	13	1.8
canned FRAY BENTOS	**198**	4.8	14.9	13.2	n/a
frozen ROSS	**295**	6.6	24.6	19.4	1
frozen, each BIRDS EYE	**470**	11	43	28	3.2
canned TYNE BRAND	**161**	8.7	13.3	8.1	n/a
Pork Pie, individual	**363**	10.8	23.7	25.7	n/a
Pork & Egg Pie (Gala)	**314**	14	15	22	2.3
Quiche Lorraine, recipe	**358**	13.7	19.6	25.5	n/a
Quiche					
cheese & egg, recipe	**315**	12.4	17.1	22.3	n/a
three cheese & spring onion	**237**	9	12	17	0.4

All amounts per 100g/100ml unless otherwise stated	Cal kcal	Pro g	Carb g	Fat g	Fibre g
Sausage Rolls					
flaky pastry	**383**	9.9	25.4	27.6	n/a
short pastry ROSS	**289**	11.1	19.4	19.3	0.8
vegetarian LINDA MCCARTNEY FOODS	**260**	10.9	23.1	14.5	1.6
Steak Pie, individual	**298**	9	25	18	1.1
Steak & Ale Pie, canned FRAY BENTOS	**187**	7.3	13.3	11.7	n/a
Steak & Kidney Deep Pie, frozen, family ROSS	**270**	7.2	23.9	16.7	1
Steak & Kidney Pie					
canned FRAY BENTOS	**169**	7.7	11.8	10.1	n/a
canned PRINCE'S	**179**	8.8	14.8	9.4	n/a
individual	**298**	8	26	18	0.9
frozen, each BIRDS EYE	**490**	13	38	32	2.8
frozen, individual ROSS	**232**	8.5	22.4	12.4	0.9
pastry top only	**286**	15.2	15.9	18.4	0.6
Steak & Kidney Pudding, canned FRAY BENTOS	**225**	8	20.7	12.3	n/a
Steak & Mushroom Pie, canned FRAY BENTOS	**182**	6.7	13.2	11.3	n/a
Vegetable Pie, frozen ROSS	**246**	5.1	27.5	13.9	2.5
Yorkshire Pudding, medium, frozen	**241**	9	31	9	2.4

READY MEALS (FROZEN, TINNED OR FRESH)

All amounts per 100g/100ml unless otherwise stated	Cal kcal	Pro g	Carb g	Fat g	Fibre g
TRADITIONAL					
Beef & Kidney TYNE BRAND	97	10.5	2	5.2	n/a
Beef Casserole TYNE BRAND	93	6.2	6.5	4.7	n/a
Beef Stew recipe	107	12	4.7	4.6	n/a
CAMPBELL'S	71	4.5	8.2	2.2	n/a
Beef Stew, Spicy TYNE BRAND	106	7.5	8.1	5.1	n/a
Beef Stew & Dumpling, each					
BIRDS EYE	320	18	42	8.8	3.8
Braised Beef TYNE BRAND	102	10.9	3.2	5.1	n/a
Bubble & Squeak ROSS	111	1.7	13.8	6	1.3
Cheese & Potato Bake TYNE BRAND	93	3.4	10.6	4.1	n/a
Cheesey Pasta, made up KRAFT	235	6.1	26.5	11.5	1.1
Chicken & Broccoli Pasta Bake, each FINDUS	450	24	39	22	n/a
Chicken Casserole TYNE BRAND	100	4.2	7.1	6.3	n/a
Chicken Chargrills BIRDS EYE					
original	208	22.2	2.5	12.1	0.1
Garlic	207	22.3	3.1	11.7	0.1
Honey & Mustard Chicken	180	19.6	4.2	9.4	0.1
Thai chicken	208	20.9	4.4	11.9	0.2

All amounts per 100g/100ml unless otherwise stated	Cal kcal	Pro g	Carb g	Fat g	Fibre g
Chicken Fillet Strips with					
Dijon Mustard BIRDS EYE	**137**	18.9	3.7	5.2	0.1
Chicken Hotpot WEIGHT WATCHERS	**84**	5.4	10.1	2.4	0.7
Chicken Kiev, frozen	**294**	13	11	22	0.6
low fat	**207**	13	14	11	0.7
garlic & herb BIRDS EYE	**192**	15.5	9.9	10	2
Chicken in a Creamy Mushroom					
Sauce WEIGHT WATCHERS	**95**	6.5	11.1	2.7	0.6
Chicken in a mushroom & Herb					
Sauce, frozen WEIGHT WATCHERS	**76**	87	4	2.8	1
Chicken Ravioli in a Spicy					
Indian Sauce HEINZ	**81**	2.8	13.7	1.6	0.5
Chicken Stew CAMPBELL'S	**69**	3.6	7.5	2.8	n/a
Chicken Stew & Dumplings,					
each BIRDS EYE	**310**	22	37	8	4.2
Chicken Supreme with Rice					
WEIGHT WATCHERS	**85**	5.5	11.7	1.7	0.5
each BIRDS EYE	**470**	25	71	9.8	1.9
Chunky Chicken Supreme,					
canned SHIPPAMS	**159**	13	4.5	10.1	n/a-
Chunky Chicken Curry,					
canned SHIPPAMS	**121**	12	4.6	6.2	n/a
Cottage Pie ROSS	**75**	3	10.9	2.2	0.3

All amounts per 100g/100ml unless otherwise stated	Cal kcal	Pro g	Carb g	Fat g	Fibre g
Cracked Pepper Chicken					
BIRDS EYE	**206**	21	3.9	11.8	0.1
Crispy Chicken BIRDS EYE	**236**	15	10.2	15	0.3
Faggots	**268**	11.1	15.3	18.5	N
in a rich West Country sauce					
MR BRAIN'S	**125**	6.5	11.3	6	0.9
Irish Stew recipe	**118**	7.4	8.6	6.2	n/a
BUMPER HARVEST	**87**	3.7	8.8	4.1	n/a
Lancashire Hotpot recipe	**119**	7.4	7.4	6.9	n/a
TYNE BRAND	**77**	4.5	7.2	3.3	n/a
Macaroni Cheese recipe	**162**	6.7	12.2	9.9	n/a
canned HEINZ	**84**	3.8	11	2.8	0.3
frozen FINDUS	**150**	5.5	16	7	0.4
frozen ROSS	**109**	4.2	16.2	3.1	1.3
Mince & Vegetables, Farmhouse					
TYNE BRAND	**74**	5.9	6.7	2.6	n/a
Minced Beef & Onion TYNE BRAND	**115**	9.5	7	5.5	n/a
Pepper Steak, Meal for One,					
each CHICAGO TOWN	**384**	17	52.1	12	n/a
Roast Beef Dinner, each BIRDS EYE	**385**	31	44	9.3	5
in gravy, pack BIRDS EYE	**120**	15	3.6	4.8	0.1
Roast Chicken Dinner, each					
BIRDS EYE	**475**	37	46	16	5

All amounts per 100g/100ml unless otherwise stated	Cal kcal	Pro g	Carb g	Fat g	Fibre g
Roast Lamb Dinner, each					
BIRDS EYE	**400**	26	45	13	5
Roast Pork Dinner, each BIRDS EYE	**410**	26	50	12	5.4
Roast Turkey Dinner, each					
BIRDS EYE	**395**	24	47	12	5
Savoury Mince TYNE BRAND	**86**	9.8	13.4	7.3	0.6
Shepherd's Pie BIRDS EYE	**85**	4.5	11.5	2.3	1.2
WEIGHT WATCHERS	**73**	3.5	10.1	2.1	0.9
vegetarian LINDA MCCARTNEY FOODS	**84**	3.7	12.3	2.2	2.3
Spicy Meatballs, Meal for One,					
each CHICAGO TOWN	**471**	13.6	66	17	n/a
Stewed Steak with Gravy	**158**	16.2	0.6	10.1	n/a
Vegetable Casserole, frozen ROSS	**96**	3.4	15.4	2.3	2
Vegetable Hotpot WEIGHT WATCHERS	**68**	2.6	9.9	1.9	1.5

CHINESE

Chinese Chicken & Prawn Foo					
Yeung Stir Fry ROSS	**77**	5.5	12.3	1.4	1.8
Chinese Chicken Stir Fry ROSS	**57**	5.7	9.6	0.8	2.8
Chinese Prawns Stir Fry ROSS	**60**	3.3	12.4	0.4	1.5
Chinese Sizzling Prawns Stir Fry					
ROSS	**39**	3.3	8.2	0.3	2.5

All amounts per 100g/100ml unless otherwise stated	Cal kcal	Pro g	Carb g	Fat g	Fibre g
Chinese Spring Rolls Ross	114	4	22.5	1.6	1.7
Chinese Sweet & Sour Pork Stir Fry Ross	63	4.1	12	0.8	2.1
Chow Mein, as sold Vesta	318	14.8	54	4.7	7.7
Oriental Chicken, each Birds Eye	335	28	36	8.8	1.2
Sweet Chilli Chicken Birds Eye	225	14.4	18.7	10.3	0.8
Sweet Chilli Noodles, Wok Findus	100	3	20	0.5	n/a

ITALIAN

	Cal kcal	Pro g	Carb g	Fat g	Fibre g
Bolognese Shells Italiana canned Weight Watchers	71	5.2	9.6	1.3	0.8
Bolognese Sauce with Beef Campbell's	58	2.5	8.9	1.4	n/a
Chicken & Broccoli Pasta Bake Weight Watchers	92	6.4	11	2.5	0.7
Chicken & Red Wine Penne canned Weight Watchers	63	3.7	10.1	0.7	0.6
Chicken Arrabiatta, Pasta Presto, each Findus	75	5.5	11	2	n/a
Chicken Fillet Strips with Red Pesto Birds Eye	135	19.1	3.2	5.1	0.2

All amounts per 100g/100ml unless otherwise stated	Cal kcal	Pro g	Carb g	Fat g	Fibre g
Chicken in Pesto Sauce, each					
BIRDS EYE	**440**	34	40	16	5.2
Chicken in Tomato & Basil					
Sauce, each BIRDS EYE	**400**	36	49	6.4	2.4
Lasagne					
recipe	**191**	9.8	14.6	10.8	n/a
beef, each BIRDS EYE	**490**	23	52	21	2.8
beef, Pasta Presto FINDUS	**100**	6	12	3	n/a
beef WEIGHT WATCHERS	**96**	6.3	9.7	3.4	0.3
chicken, leek & mushroom					
Pasta Presto FINDUS	**110**	5.5	13	4	n/a
frozen, cooked	**143**	7.4	15.7	6.1	n/a
vegetable, Pasta Presto FINDUS	**80**	3	12	2.5	n/a
vegetable ROSS	**110**	5.3	12.6	4.7	0.9
vegetable WEIGHT WATCHERS	**78**	3.2	12.9	1.5	1
Mediterranean Chicken BIRDS EYE	**240**	14.6	16	13.1	1
Mexican Lasagne, Pasta Presto					
FINDUS	**110**	6	13	3	n/a
Penne Napoletana, Pasta					
Presto FINDUS	**80**	2.5	13	2.5	n/a
Ravioli, Italiana, vegetable with					
tomato sauce, WEIGHT WATCHERS	**69**	1.7	10.9	2.1	0.5
Risotto	**233**	3.5	35.1	9.7	n/a
beef, as sold VESTA	**346**	15.3	57.8	5.9	5.6
chicken & lemon	**98**	5.9	12.5	2.8	0.5

All amounts per 100g/100ml unless otherwise stated	Cal kcal	Pro g	Carb g	Fat g	Fibre g
Spaghetti Bolognese					
each BIRDS EYE	**445**	26	60	11	3.7
frozen, as sold ROSS	**90**	4.2	15.7	1.1	0.9
Pasta Presto, each FINDUS	**380**	18	63	6.5	4
Spicy Sausage Penne Pasta,					
Pasta Presto FINDUS	**95**	3.5	11	4	n/a
Spinach & Ricotta Cannelloni,					
frozen ROSS	**107**	3.7	16.7	2.8	2
Sundried Tomato, Mascarpone &					
Chicken Spiralli, Pasta Presto					
FINDUS	**90**	4.5	12	3	n/a
Tagliatelle					
Carbonara WEIGHT WATCHERS	**88**	5.3	12.2	2	0.4
Spinach, bacon & mushroom,					
Pasta Presto FINDUS	**120**	5	17	4	n/a
Tomato & Basil Chicken with					
Potato Wedges WEIGHT WATCHERS	**74**	4.6	9.1	2.1	1
Tortellini					
Italiana WEIGHT WATCHERS	**62**	2	9.4	1.8	0.6
Spicy Italiana WEIGHT WATCHERS	**60**	2.8	9.9	1	0.9
Tortelloni DOLMIO					
with 4 cheeses	**187**	7.6	22.1	7.6	n/a
with ham & cheese	**183**	7.4	22.2	7.1	n/a
with sun-dried tomato & cheese	**187**	7.4	23.8	6.9	n/a
Tuscan Chicken WEIGHT WATCHERS	**800**	8.7	5.8	2.5	1

All amounts per 100g/100ml unless otherwise stated	Cal kcal	Pro g	Carb g	Fat g	Fibre g
INDIAN					
Beef Curry					
FINDUS	**130**	5	21	3	0.8
TYNE BRAND	**98**	5.5	9.2	4.3	n/a
per meal VESTA	**927**	30.6	157.2	19.5	13.4
Beef Curry with Rice, pack					
BIRDS EYE	**510**	23	80	11	2.9
Chicken Balti & Rice Curry					
Break PATAK	**90**	4.7	11.6	2.8	n/a
Chicken Curry					
FINDUS	**120**	6	19	2.5	0.6
TYNE BRAND	**149**	4.5	11	9.7	n/a
Chicken Curry, Creamy COLMAN'S	**392**	10.8	51.2	16	6.6
Chicken Curry with Rice					
pack BIRDS EYE	**500**	24	78	10	2.5
frozen, as sold ROSS	**85**	3.4	14.7	1.3	0.5
WEIGHT WATCHERS	**91**	4.8	14.3	1.7	0.5
Chicken Jalfrezi with Basmati					
Rice WEIGHT WATCHERS	**72**	5	11.8	0.5	0.5
Chicken Korma with Rice					
WEIGHT WATCHERS	**97**	5.8	13.5	2.1	0.2
Chicken Tikka Balti					
WEIGHT WATCHERS	**71**	4.2	10	1.6	0.7

All amounts per 100g/100ml unless otherwise stated	Cal kcal	Pro g	Carb g	Fat g	Fibre g
Chicken Tikka Masala Curry Break PATAK	152	5.8	12.7	8.6	n/a
Chicken Tikka Masala with Rice, pack BIRDS EYE	490	22	74	12	2.5
Curried Beef & Vegetables TYNE BRAND	87	3.7	11	3.4	n/a
Curried Mince & Vegetables TYNE BRAND	100	5.7	9.6	4.3	n/a
Indian Chicken Stir Fry Meal ROSS	74	5.8	15.2	0.6	3.7
Lamb Curry TYNE BRAND	99	6.1	7.2	5.1	n/a
Prawn Curry with rice ROSS	86	2.9	15.7	1.3	1
Prawn Curry with Rice, pack BIRDS EYE	485	16	76	13	2.1
Samosas meat	272	11.4	18.9	17.3	N
vegetable	217	5.1	30	9.3	n/a
Vegetable Curry TYNE BRAND	57	2	9.6	1.4	n/a
Vegetable Tikka Masala Curry Break PATAK	112	2.4	13.6	5.4	n/a

All amounts per 100g/100ml unless otherwise stated	Cal kcal	Pro g	Carb g	Fat g	Fibre g
MEXICAN					
Burrito Dinner Kit OLD EL PASO					
salsa	**28**	1	6	0	n/a
spice mix	**304**	13	54	4	n/a
tortilla	**343**	10	60	7	n/a
Chicken Mexicana with Rice					
WEIGHT WATCHERS	**97**	5.8	13.5	2.1	0.2
Chilli Con Carne TYNE BRAND	**106**	9.4	6.6	4.7	n/a
Chilli Con Carne, each BIRDS EYE	**290**	9.4	47	7.1	2.3
Chilli with Beans & Vegetables					
TYNE BRAND	**111**	5.9	12.5	4.2	n/a
Enchilada Dinner Kit OLD EL PASO					
spice mix	**303**	8	52	7	n/a
tom sauce	**56**	2	12	0	n/a
tortilla	**343**	10	60	7	n/a
Fajita Dinner Kit OLD EL PASO					
salsa	**28**	1	6	0	n/a
spice mix	**306**	9	54	6	n/a
tortilla	**343**	10	60	7	n/a
Fajita Dinner Kit, Roasted					
Tomato & Peppers OLD EL PASO					
salsa	**37**	1.3	8	0.5	n/a
spice mix	**277**	66	55.6	3.1	n/a
tortilla	**323**	9	52	9	n/a

All amounts per 100g/100ml unless otherwise stated	Cal kcal	Pro g	Carb g	Fat g	Fibre g
Fajita Chicken Wrap					
CHICAGO TOWN	**217**	8.6	27.1	8.2	1
Mexican Chilli with Deep Fried					
Potato Wedges WEIGHT WATCHERS	**84**	5.1	10.3	2.5	1.7
Taco Dinner Kit OLD EL PASO					
salsa	**40**	1	9	0	n/a
spice mix	**336**	6	69	4	n/a
taco shells	**506**	7	61	26	n/a
Spicy Mexican Chicken BIRDS EYE	**236**	14.6	16.3	12.5	0.9
WORLD					
Caribbean Chicken Stir Fry ROSS	**88**	5.9	13.8	1.7	1.5
Japanese Beef Oriental Stir Fry					
ROSS	**62**	5.4	9.4	1	1.5
Spicy Lamb Kebabs ROSS	**298**	13.9	3.6	25.5	1
Lemon Pepper Chicken BIRDS EYE	**243**	14.8	19.1	11.9	0.7
Moussaka	**140**	8.3	8.6	8.3	n/a
lamb WEIGHT WATCHERS	**79**	3.6	10.9	2.3	0.8
Paella					
per meal VESTA	**510**	17.5	102.2	3.5	5.2
fast cook ROSS	**93**	5.6	15.6	1.4	0.9

All amounts per 100g/100ml unless otherwise stated	Cal kcal	Pro g	Carb g	Fat g	Fibre g
Southern Fried Chicken BIRDS EYE	**257**	15.1	16.5	14.5	0.7
Thai Chicken, each BIRDS EYE	**380**	27	51	7.6	3.6
Vegetable Stroganoff WEIGHT WATCHERS	**85**	2.2	15	1.9	0.6

RICE & NOODLES

All amounts per 100g/100ml unless otherwise stated	Cal kcal	Pro g	Carb g	Fat g	Fibre g
PLAIN RICE COOKED					
White Rice boiled	**138**	2.6	30.9	1.3	0.1
Easy Cook, boiled	**138**	2.6	30.9	1.3	n/a
Brown Rice, boiled	**141**	2.6	32.1	1.1	n/a
PRE-COOKED RICE					
Basmati Rice					
PATAK	**151**	2.7	29.8	2.3	n/a
Boil in the Bag UNCLE BEN'S	**343**	9	76	0.6	1.9
Express UNCLE BEN'S	**148**	3.2	30	1.7	0.5
Chinese Special Rice, frozen ROSS	**99**	4.1	21.1	0.3	1
Chinese Rice, Express UNCLE BEN'S	**156**	3.4	30.7	2.2	0.8
Coconut Flavoured Rice with Mustard Seed PATAK	**174**	2.9	30.1	4.25	n/a
Egg Fried Rice, recipe	**208**	4.2	25.7	10.6	0.4
Express UNCLE BEN'S	**173**	4	29.9	4.2	0.3
Wok FINDUS	**110**	3	21	1.5	n/a
Fried White Rice, recipe	**144**	2.5	25.9	4.1	n/a
Garlic & Coriander Flavoured Rice PATAK	**149**	2.6	28.9	2.2	n/a
Express UNCLE BEN'S	**156**	3.2	31.4	1.9	0.5
Golden Vegetable Express Rice UNCLE BEN'S	**148**	3.3	29.7	1.8	0.6

All amounts per 100g/100ml unless otherwise stated	Cal kcal	Pro g	Carb g	Fat g	Fibre g
Indian Special Rice, frozen ROSS	118	2.8	26.1	0.8	1.3
Lemon & Rosemary Express Rice UNCLE BEN'S	156	3.2	31.2	2	0.4
Long Grain & Wild Rice Boil in the Bag UNCLE BEN'S	342	8.5	74.8	1	2.6
Long Grain Rice, Boil in the Bag					
UNCLE BEN'S	346	6.3	79	0.5	1.2
Express UNCLE BEN'S	146	3	31.1	1	0.3
Mexican Express Rice UNCLE BEN'S	157	3.2	35	1.8	1
Mushroom Express Rice UNCLE BEN'S	157	3.2	31.7	1.9	0.5
Original Vegetable Rice, frozen BIRDS EYE	100	4	20.2	0.3	1.7
Pilau Rice PATAK	152	2.8	30.5	2.3	n/a
Express UNCLE BEN'S	164	3.2	30.8	3.1	0.9
Savoury Rice, cooked	142	2.9	26.3	3.5	n/a
Sweet & Spicy Express Rice UNCLE BEN'S	169	2.7	30.5	4	0.8
Tomato & Basil Express Rice UNCLE BEN'S	181	3.5	32.2	4.2	0.6
Vegetable Pilau Express Rice UNCLE BEN'S	156	3	29	3.1	0.6

All amounts per 100g/100ml unless otherwise stated	Cal kcal	Pro g	Carb g	Fat g	Fibre g

DRY RICE

Arborio Risotto Rice	350	7.4	77.5	1.1	1.1
Arrosito Seasoned Rice					
OLD EL PASO	357	9	78	1	n/a
Basmati Rice					
UNCLE BEN'S	343	9	76	0.6	1.9
WHITWORTHS	339	7.4	79.8	0.5	0.5
Beef Savoury Rice BATCHELORS	359	8.9	75.7	2.3	2.5
Chinese Savoury Rice BATCHELORS	359	9.4	75.5	2.2	2.1
Chicken Savoury Rice BATCHELORS	367	8.9	79.4	1.5	2.6
Egg Fried Rice BATCHELORS	369	8.6	77.9	2.6	1.3
Garlic Butter Savoury Rice					
BATCHELORS	370	8.6	78.7	2.3	1.9
Golden Savoury Rice BATCHELORS	366	9.3	78.9	1.5	4.5
Long Grain Rice					
UNCLE BEN'S	346	6.3	79	0.5	1.2
WHITWORTHS	361	6.5	86.8	1	0.5
Long Grain & Wild Rice					
UNCLE BEN'S	347	11.2	92.8	1.2	n/a
Mild Curry Savoury Rice					
BATCHELORS	355	8	76.1	2.1	1.6

All amounts per 100g/100ml unless otherwise stated	Cal kcal	Pro g	Carb g	Fat g	Fibre g
Mushroom Savoury Rice BATCHELORS	**356**	10.7	73.6	2.1	2.8
Pudding Rice	**355**	6.3	80.5	0.9	0.5
Risotto Rice WHITWORTHS	**324**	7	77.8	0.6	0.2
Short Grain Rice WHITWORTHS	**361**	6.5	86.8	1	2.4
Wholegrain Rice UNCLE BEN'S	**336**	8	71	2.2	4.7
NOODLES, COOKED					
Egg Noodles, boiled	**62**	2.2	13	0.5	n/a
DRY NOODLES					
Egg Noodles, fine SHARWOOD	**346**	12	70	2.1	2.5
Egg Noodles, medium SHARWOOD	**346**	12	70	2.1	2.5
Rice Noodles SHARWOOD	**382**	6.5	86.8	1	2.4
Stir Fry Noodles SHARWOOD	**170**	5.4	32.5	2	3.1
Thread Noodles AMOY	**169**	6	24.5	5.2	n/a

SAVOURY SPREADS & PASTES

All amounts per 100g/100ml unless otherwise stated	Cal kcal	Pro g	Carb g	Fat g	Fibre g
Anchovy Paste SHIPPAMS	**137**	19.7	3.2	5	n/a
Beef Paste	**194**	17	0.1	14	Tr
Beef Pâté SHIPPAMS	**204**	17.3	1.5	14.3	n/a
Bloater Pâté SHIPPAMS	**172**	18	2.2	10.1	n/a
Cheese Spread	**267**	11.3	4.4	22.8	0
KERRYGOLD	**213**	n/a	8.5	15	0
reduced fat	**175**	15	7.9	9.5	0

See also: **DAIRY PRODUCTS (Cheese spreads & processed cheese)**

	Cal kcal	Pro g	Carb g	Fat g	Fibre g
Chicken & Ham Pâté SHIPPAMS	**226**	15.6	1.3	17.6	n/a
Chicken & Mayonnaise-style Dressing Sandwich Filler HEINZ	**191**	6.3	7.7	15	0.3
Chicken in Curry Mayonnaise Sandwich Maker SHIPPAMS	**206**	13.1	2.3	16.1	n/a
Chicken in Mayonnaise Sandwich Maker SHIPPAMS	**213**	113	2.3	16.9	n/a
Chicken Paste	**184**	16	0.8	13	0.7
Chicken Pâté SHIPPAMS	**233**	14.7	1.6	18.6	n/a
Chicken Tikka & Mayonnaise Pâté SHIPPAMS	**273**	15.7	4.6	21.3	n/a
Crab Pâté SHIPPAMS	**96**	15.9	1.2	3.1	n/a
luxury Orkney CASTLE MACLELLAN	**171**	10.7	5.9	11.6	0.4

All amounts per 100g/100ml unless otherwise stated	Cal kcal	Pro g	Carb g	Fat g	Fibre g
Curried Chicken Sandwich Filler					
HEINZ	**192**	6.2	9.6	14.2	0.7
Fish Paste	**170**	15.3	3.7	10.5	n/a
Ham Sandwich Filler HEINZ	**198**	5.4	11	14.7	0.5
Marmite Yeast Extract MARMITE	**231**	38.4	19.2	0.1	3.1
Prawn & Salad Vegetables Sandwich Filler HEINZ	**129**	4.4	9.5	8.1	0.6
Salmon & Shrimp Pâté SHIPPAMS	**182**	15.3	2.4	12.4	n/a
Sandwich Spread HEINZ	**221**	1.3	25.3	12.7	0.8
cucumber	**185**	1.3	18.9	11.5	0.5
Smoked Salmon Pâté, Scottish CASTLE MACLELLAN	**278**	12.2	3.4	23.9	0.4
Toast Topper HEINZ					
chicken & mushroom	**56**	5.1	5.7	1.4	0.2
ham & cheese	**96**	7.4	7.3	4.1	0.1
mushroom & bacon	**94**	6.9	6.6	4.4	0.3
Tuna Sandwich Filler HEINZ	**192**	6.3	11.7	13.4	0.3
Carb Check HEINZ	**161**	6.6	6.3	12	0.7
Vegemite KRAFT	**191**	25.6	19.5	0.9	0

SNACK MEALS

All amounts per 100g/100ml unless otherwise stated	Cal kcal	Pro g	Carb g	Fat g	Fibre g
Bacon Sizzler Pot Noodle, as prepared POT NOODLE COMPANY	**116**	2.3	15.5	4.9	1.1
Bacon Supernoodles BATCHELORS	**457**	9.8	60.9	19.7	3.2
Balti Pot Curry POT NOODLE COMPANY	**89**	3.1	17.8	0.5	0.5
Barbecue Beef Supernoodles BATCHELORS	**451**	9.4	60.6	19.7	3.2
BBQ Micro Ribs MCCAIN	**234**	18.7	7.2	14.7	n/a
BBQ Noodles PEPERAMI	**477**	10.3	57.6	22.7	2.1
Beef & Tomato Mini Pot Noodle, as prepared POT NOODLE COMPANY	**134**	3.5	18.7	5	1.7
Beef & Tomato Pot Noodle, as prepared POT NOODLE COMPANY	**126**	3.1	18.1	4.7	1.1
Beef Ciabatta MCCAIN	**276**	10.6	30.9	12.3	n/a
Bombay Bad Boy Pot Noodle, as prepared POT NOODLE COMPANY	**126**	3	16.9	5.2	1.1
Cajun Micro Wings MCCAIN	**226**	21.8	3.8	13.7	n/a
Chargrilled Chicken Salad Sandwich WEIGHT WATCHERS	**153**	9.4	17.7	4.9	2.1
Cheese & Ham Micro Toastie MCCAIN	**282**	10	36	10.9	n/a
Cheese & Ham Supernoodles BATCHELORS	**472**	9.4	63.2	20.2	1.5

All amounts per 100g/100ml unless otherwise stated	Cal kcal	Pro g	Carb g	Fat g	Fibre g
Cheese & Onion Micro Toastie McCAIN	**273**	8.2	35.6	10.8	n/a
Cheese & Pepperoni New Snack Stop CROSSE & BLACKWELL	**100**	2.9	13.3	4.1	0.4
Chicken & Herb Supernoodles 98% fat free BATCHELORS	**342**	11	71.5	1.3	2.6
Chicken & Mushroom Mini Pot, as prepared POT NOODLE COMPANY	**128**	3.8	18.2	4.5	1.4
Chicken & Mushroom Pot Noodle, as prepared POT NOODLE COMPANY	**128**	3.2	18	4.7	1.1
Chicken & Sweetcorn New Snack Stop CROSSE & BLACKWELL	**100**	2.7	13.8	3.9	0.5
Chicken Balti Filled Naans PATAK	**243**	6.2	35.2	8.6	3.2
Chicken Ciabatta McCAIN	**208**	14.1	27.1	4.8	n/a
Chicken Snack Pot, Italian Style, Carb Check HEINZ	**60**	5.9	4.3	2	1
Chicken Supernoodles BATCHELORS	**449**	8.7	60.3	19.2	2.5
Chicken Tikka Naan McCAIN	**223**	8.9	31.3	6.9	n/a
Chicken Tikka Sandwich WEIGHT WATCHERS	**177**	13.1	21.4	4.4	1.5
Chinese Chow Mein Supernoodles BATCHELORS	**458**	9.2	60.5	19.8	2.9

All amounts per 100g/100ml unless otherwise stated	Cal kcal	Pro g	Carb g	Fat g	Fibre g
Chinese Micro Ribs McCAIN	**258**	19.1	7.7	16.8	n/a
Chinese Micro Wings McCAIN	**213**	18.1	7	12.5	n/a
Chow Mein Pot Noodle, as prepared POT NOODLE COMPANY	**127**	3	18	4.8	1.1
Cumberland Sausage & Onion Baguette McCAIN	**259**	11.1	36.1	7.8	n/a
Dairylea Lunchables each KRAFT					
chicken	**320**	19	19.5	18	0.8
ham	**325**	18.5	20	18	0.8
hotdog	**280**	12.5	18.5	17	0.6
Egg Salad Sandwich with Salad Cream WEIGHT WATCHERS	**155**	6.9	21	4.8	0.9
Flips FINDUS					
cheese & ham	**170**	6.5	25	4.5	n/a
chilli beef	**160**	7	23	4.5	n/a
Fried Chicken Noodles PEPERAMI	**477**	10.3	57.6	22.7	2.1
Ham & Cheese Pasta New Snack Stop CROSSE & BLACKWELL	**115**	4	15.5	4	0.1
Hot & Spicy Noodles PEPERAMI	**476**	10.3	58.5	22.3	2.3
Korma Pot Curry, as prepared POT NOODLE COMPANY	**91**	2.9	17.4	1	0.4
Tuna Snack Pot, Carb Check HEINZ Breton Style	**109**	8.4	4.6	6.3	1.5

All amounts per 100g/100ml unless otherwise stated	Cal kcal	Pro g	Carb g	Fat g	Fibre g
Mediterranean Style	**68**	8.2	4.8	1.8	1.4
Micro Noodles, as prepared KNORR					
chicken flavour	**178**	3.6	21.6	8.4	1
chow mein flavour	**176**	3.5	21.9	8.2	0.7
mild curry flavour	**179**	3.3	22.2	8.5	0.8
Mild Curry Supernoodles BATCHELORS	**457**	9.5	60.6	19.7	3
Mild Mexican Chilli Supernoodles, as served BATCHELORS	**175**	3.1	23.2	7.8	0.5
Mushroom Supernoodles BATCHELORS	**454**	9.3	60.5	19.7	3
Nice 'n' Spicy Pot Noodle, as prepared POT NOODLE COMPANY	**127**	2.8	18.3	4.7	1.1
Original Noodles PEPERAMI	**476**	10.3	58.5	22.3	2.3
Pepperoni, Mozzarella & Tomato Panini MCCAIN	**259**	11.6	30.5	10.1	n/a
Prawn Cocktail Sandwich WEIGHT WATCHERS	**145**	8.9	16.6	4.8	2.5
Roast Onion & Potato New Snack Stop CROSSE & BLACKWELL	**100**	1.7	14.4	3.7	0.6
Roast Parsnip & Potato New Snack Stop CROSSE & BLACKWELL	**95**	1.7	13.6	3.6	1.1

All amounts per 100g/100ml unless otherwise stated	Cal kcal	Pro g	Carb g	Fat g	Fibre g
Saucy BBQ Pasta New Snack Stop CROSSE & BLACKWELL	**95**	2.6	17.5	0.8	0.2
Seedy Sanchez Pot Noodle, as prepared POT NOODLE COMPANY	**132**	3.1	19.1	4.8	1.1
Smoked Ham & 4 Cheeses Panini MCCAIN	**280**	13.6	31.8	10.9	n/a
Soft Cheese & Roasted Peppers Sandwich, low fat WEIGHT WATCHERS	**181**	9.7	27	3.9	1.5
Southern Fried Chicken Supernoodles BATCHELORS	**471**	9.2	64.1	19.8	1.4
Spag Bol Supernoodles BATCHELORS	**470**	9	64.5	19.5	1.5
Spicy Chilli Posh Noodle, as prepared POT NOODLE COMPANY	**112**	1.8	15.6	4.7	0.5
Spicy Chinese Chicken Posh Noodle, as prepared POT NOODLE COMPANY	**111**	1.8	17.2	3.9	0.6
Spicy Curry Pot Noodle, as prepared POT NOODLE COMPANY	**131**	2.9	19.1	4.8	1.1
Spicy Thai Chilli Supernoodles 98% fat free BATCHELORS	**343**	10.6	72.5	1.2	3
Spicy Tomato Pasta New Snack Stop CROSSE & BLACKWELL	**87**	2.4	15.9	1.5	0.2

All amounts per 100g/100ml unless otherwise stated	Cal kcal	Pro g	Carb g	Fat g	Fibre g
Sweet & Sour Posh Noodle, as prepared POT NOODLE COMPANY	125	1.7	19.2	4.6	0.5
Sweet & Sour Pot Noodle, as prepared POT NOODLE COMPANY	126	2.7	18	4.8	1.1
Sweet & Sour Supernoodles BATCHELORS	455	8.8	60.8	19.7	3.1
Take Out Curry Pasta New Snack Stop CROSSE & BLACKWELL	100	2.7	16.9	2.1	0.5
Tikka Masala Pot Curry, as prepared POT NOODLE COMPANY	82	3.1	17.5	0.8	0.3
Tomato & Ham Pasta New Snack Stop CROSSE & BLACKWELL	100	3.1	16.8	2.1	0.2
Tomato & Herb New Snack Stop CROSSE & BLACKWELL	85	2.6	16.1	1.1	0.5
Tuna Salad Sandwich WEIGHT WATCHERS	137	10.5	13.9	4.4	2.4
Tuna, Sweetcorn & Montery Jack Cheese Baguette MCCAIN	247	12.1	34.3	6.8	n/a

SOUPS

All amounts per 100g/100ml unless otherwise stated	Cal kcal	Pro g	Carb g	Fat g	Fibre g
American Potato & Leek Soup of the World, as sold KNORR	359	8.1	58.3	10.4	5.7
Austrian Cream of Herb Soup of the World, as sold KNORR	464	9.1	42.7	28.5	2.2
Autumn Vegetable Soup BAXTERS	48	2.2	9.2	0.3	1.5
Beef Broth HEINZ BIG SOUPS	43	2.2	6.9	0.7	1
Beef Consommé BAXTERS	13	2.6	0.7	Tr	0
Beef & Tomato Cup-A-Soup, per sachet BATCHELORS	83	1.4	15.8	1.6	1
Beef & Vegetable Soup HEINZ BIG SOUPS	48	2.9	7.2	0.8	1
Broccoli & Cauliflower Slim-A-Soup, per sachet BATCHELORS	59	0.9	10	1.7	0.5
Broccoli, Stilton & Bacon Soup BAXTERS	45	1.3	5.9	1.8	0.4
Butternut Squash & Red Pepper Soup BAXTERS	36	0.7	6.1	1	0.6
Cajun Spicy Vegetable Slim-A-Soup, per sachet BATCHELORS	52	1.7	9.4	0.8	1.6
Carrot & Butter Bean Soup BAXTERS	54	1.6	7.7	1.9	1.7
Carrot & Coriander Soup BAXTERS	41	0.8	6	1.5	0.8

All amounts per 100g/100ml unless otherwise stated	Cal kcal	Pro g	Carb g	Fat g	Fibre g
as sold KNORR	**394**	6.9	50.1	18.2	6.6
Carrot & Ginger Special Soup					
HEINZ	**47**	1.1	5.3	2.4	0.8
Carrot & Lentil Soup					
WEIGHT WATCHERS	**31**	1.4	6	0.1	0.8
Carrot, Onion & Chick Pea Soup					
BAXTERS	**41**	1.8	7.7	0.3	1
Carrot, Potato & Coriander Soup					
WEIGHT WATCHERS	**24**	0.5	5.4	0.1	0.6
Carrot with Crème Fraiche Soup					
BAXTERS	**41**	0.5	5.9	1.7	0.7
Chargrilled Chicken & White Wine with Shallots Soup BAXTERS	**84**	2.8	5.9	5.5	0.1
Cheese & Broccoli Cup-A-Soup Extra, per sachet BATCHELORS	**160**	5.2	23.5	5	1.9
Chicken & Leek Cup-A-Soup, per sachet BATCHELORS	**96**	1.2	12.2	4.7	1.7
Chicken & Mushroom					
CAMPBELL'S	**56**	0.8	3.5	4.3	n/a
Cup-A-Soup Extra, per sachet BATCHELORS	**132**	3.7	20.2	4	1.3
Slim-A-Soup, per sachet BATCHELORS	**60**	1.3	9	2.1	0.9

All amounts per 100g/100ml unless otherwise stated	Cal kcal	Pro g	Carb g	Fat g	Fibre g
Chicken & Sweetcorn Slim-A-Soup, per sachet BATCHELORS	**55**	1.2	8.5	1.8	0.9
Chicken & Vegetable Broth with Rice GRANNY'S	**46**	0.5	6.9	1.8	n/a
Chicken & Vegetable Cup-A-Soup, per sachet					
BATCHELORS	**137**	1.3	18	6.6	2.2
BAXTERS	**36**	1.7	6.1	0.5	1.2
HEINZ BIG SOUPS	**47**	2.9	7.4	0.6	0.9
Chicken & White Wine Soup, diluted CAMPBELL'S	**47**	0.9	3.8	3.2	n/a
Chicken Broth BAXTERS	**31**	1.5	5.4	0.4	0.6
Chunky Chilled Soup BAXTERS	**35**	2.1	4	1.2	0.7
Chicken Consommé BAXTERS	**10**	1.1	0.8	Tr	0
Chicken Cup-A-Soup, per sachet					
BATCHELORS	**83**	1.1	8.3	5	1.4
WEIGHT WATCHERS	**30**	1.2	4.1	1	0
99% fat-free, diluted CAMPBELL'S	**25**	0.9	3.7	0.7	n/a
Chicken, Mushroom & Potato Soup HEINZ BIG SOUPS	**66**	3.4	8.1	2.3	0.4
Chicken Noodle Cup-A-Soup, per sachet					
BATCHELORS	**96**	4.3	17	1.2	0.7
GRANNY'S	**33**	0.7	5.5	0.9	n/a

All amounts per 100g/100ml unless otherwise stated	Cal kcal	Pro g	Carb g	Fat g	Fibre g
HEINZ	27	1.1	4.9	0.3	0.2
WEIGHT WATCHERS	17	0.7	3.1	0.1	0.2
as sold, super KNORR	325	14.3	56	4.8	1.8
Chicken, Noodle & Vegetable Slim-A-Soup, per sachet					
BATCHELORS	55	1.6	10	1	1.2
Chicken Pasta & Vegetable Soup					
HEINZ BIG SOUP	34	1.8	5.9	0.4	0.8
Chicken with Vegetables **Chilled Soup** BAXTERS	102	2.4	5.4	7.9	0.4
Chinese Chicken Noodle Cup-A-Soup Extra, per sachet					
BATCHELORS	101	3.5	19.1	1.2	2
Chinese Chicken Noodle Soups **of the World,** as sold KNORR	307	15.1	51.8	4.4	2.9
Chunky Country Vegetable **Chilled Soup** BAXTERS	46	1.9	8.9	0.3	1.5
Chunky Minestrone Chilled Soup					
BAXTERS	38	1.5	6.5	0.7	1.1
Cock-a-Leekie Soup BAXTERS	23	0.9	4.1	0.3	0.3
Chilled Soup BAXTERS	33	2.1	3.2	1.3	0.5
Consommé CAMPBELL'S	8	1.5	0.6	0	n/a
Country Garden Soup BAXTERS	35	0.9	6.6	0.6	0.8

All amounts per 100g/100ml unless otherwise stated	Cal kcal	Pro g	Carb g	Fat g	Fibre g
Cream of Asparagus Soup					
Cup-A-Soup, per sachet					
BATCHELORS	134	0.7	18	6.6	2.3
BAXTERS	67	1.1	6	4.3	0.2
HEINZ	46	1.1	4.5	2.6	0.2
as sold KNORR	426	8.3	54.4	19.6	1.3
diluted CAMPBELL'S	44	0.5	4.3	2.8	n/a
low carbohydrate CARB OPTIONS	37	0.7	2.9	2.6	0.5
Cream of Celery Soup					
diluted CAMPBELL'S	46	0.6	3	3.6	n/a
HEINZ	44	0.8	4.1	2.7	0.2
Cream of Chicken Soup					
BAXTERS	69	1.8	6.1	4.2	0.1
diluted CAMPBELL'S	48	1.1	3.5	3.6	n/a
HEINZ	49	1.5	4.5	2.7	0.1
as sold KNORR	481	8.9	45.8	29.2	0.3
Cream of Chicken & Mushroom Soup HEINZ	50	1.6	4.6	2.8	0.1
Cream of Mushroom Soup					
BAXTERS	63	0.9	5.5	4.1	0.1
diluted CAMPBELL'S	56	0.7	3.5	4.4	n/a
Cup-A-Soup with croutons, per sachet BATCHELORS	121	0.9	15.2	6.3	2
as sold KNORR	500	5.2	47.8	31.8	1
Cream of Sweetcorn Soup,					
diluted CAMPBELL'S	53	0.6	6.2	2.9	n/a

All amounts per 100g/100ml unless otherwise stated	Cal kcal	Pro g	Carb g	Fat g	Fibre g
Cream of Tomato Soup					
BAXTERS	76	1.4	11.6	2.7	0.6
diluted CAMPBELL'S	66	0.8	8.4	3.2	n/a
HEINZ	57	0.9	6.6	3	0.4
as sold KNORR	485	4.8	49.5	29.6	2.6
Cream of Tomato & Red Pepper Soup, diluted CAMPBELL'S	62	0.6	7.7	3.3	n/a
Cream of Vegetable Cup-A-Soup, per sachet BATCHELORS	135	1.8	17.3	6.5	2.8
Creamy Broccoli & Cauliflower Cup-A-Soup, per sachet BATCHELORS	107	1.6	13.7	5.1	2.7
Creamy Chicken & Tarragon Cup-A-Soup, per sachet BATCHELORS	116	2	13.8	5.9	2.8
Creamy Leek & Potato Cup-A-Soup, per sachet BATCHELORS	109	1.9	15.5	4.4	3
Crofters' Thick Vegetable Soup, as sold KNORR	364	10.8	52.9	12.2	3.3
Cullen Skink Soup BAXTERS	86	6.4	7.7	3.3	0.4
English Broccoli & Stilton Soups of the World, as sold KNORR	509	11.7	30.3	37.9	1.6

All amounts per 100g/100ml unless otherwise stated	Cal kcal	Pro g	Carb g	Fat g	Fibre g
Flameroast Red Pepper & Tomato Soup BAXTERS	56	0.9	6.8	2.8	0.6
Florida Spring Vegetable Soup, as sold KNORR	290	7.8	52.2	5.6	5.2
French Onion Soup BAXTERS	21	0.7	4.3	0.1	0.4
as sold KNORR	298	5.8	62.6	2.5	6.6
Golden Vegetable Cup-A-Soup, per sachet BATCHELORS	83	1.1	14.3	2.4	0.9
as sold KNORR	394	10.7	45	19	3.3
Haggis Broth BAXTERS	52	1.8	6.8	1.9	0.7
Highlander's Broth BAXTERS	49	1.9	7	1.5	0.6
Italian Bean & Pasta Soup BAXTERS	42	2	7.9	0.3	1.1
Italian Broth with Smoked Bacon BAXTERS	53	2.3	8.8	1	1.2
Italian Minestrone Soup of the World, as sold KNORR	311	11.5	57.1	4.1	7.8
Italian Tomato with Basil Soup BAXTERS	51	2.4	8.4	0.9	0.9
diluted CAMPBELL'S	68	0.8	5.4	4.8	n/a
Leek & Chicken, as sold KNORR	458	10.3	39.7	28.7	1.4
Leek & Potato Slim-A-Soup, per sachet BATCHELORS	55	0.9	9.3	1.6	1

All amounts per 100g/100ml unless otherwise stated	Cal kcal	Pro g	Carb g	Fat g	Fibre g
Lentil & Bacon Soup BAXTERS	**55**	2.9	7.8	1.3	0.8
GRANNY'S	**66**	3.1	10	1.5	n/a
Lentil & Vegetable Soup BAXTERS	**39**	2	7.1	0.3	0.9
Lentil & Vegetables Chilled Soup BAXTERS	**52**	3.2	9	0.3	1.4
Lentil Soup					
diluted CAMPBELL'S	**47**	2.6	7.7	0.6	n/a
HEINZ	**40**	2.3	7.4	0.2	1
Lobster Bisque BAXTERS	**46**	3	4.1	2	0.2
Malaysian Chicken & Sweetcorn Soups of the World, as sold					
KNORR	**370**	10.6	56.3	11.4	1.8
Mediterranean Tomato Soup					
BAXTERS	**33**	1	6.8	0.2	0.7
99% fat free, diluted CAMPBELL'S	**27**	0.4	5.7	0.2	n/a
chilled BAXTERS	**51**	1.7	7.2	1.7	1
Slim-A-Soup, per sachet					
BATCHELORS	**54**	1.1	9.6	1.2	1
Mediterranean Tomato & Vegetable Soup WEIGHT WATCHERS	**16**	0.4	3	0.3	0.4
Minestrone Soup					
BAXTERS	**34**	1.3	5.9	0.6	0.9
HEINZ	**40**	1	5.5	1.6	0.8
as sold KNORR	**292**	9.2	53.9	4.4	6.5

All amounts per 100g/100ml unless otherwise stated	Cal kcal	Pro g	Carb g	Fat g	Fibre g
Cup-A-Soup, per sachet					
BATCHELORS	**98**	1.6	16.5	2.8	1.2
Cup-A-Soup Extra, per sachet					
BATCHELORS	**123**	3.9	24.3	1.1	2.3
WEIGHT WATCHERS	**25.3**	1.3	11.1	0.4	0.7
Slim-A-Soup with croutons,					
per sachet BATCHELORS	**56**	1.3	9.9	1.2	1.3
with cream CARB OPTIONS	**37**	0.9	3.4	2.1	0.5
with Wholemeal Pasta BAXTERS	**32**	0.9	6.6	0.2	0.8
Miso	**203**	13.3	23.5	6.2	N
Instant white with tofu, sachet,					
each MITOKU	**35**	2.4	3.9	1.1	n/a
Mulligatawny Beef Curry Soup					
HEINZ	**54**	2	7.2	1.9	0.6
Mulligatawny Soup BAXTERS	**47**	5.2	7.3	0.9	0.6
Mushroom Potage BAXTERS	**77**	1.5	6.1	5.2	0.3
Mushroom Soup WEIGHT WATCHERS	**27**	1	4.4	0.6	0.1
99% fat-free, diluted CAMPBELL'S	**24**	0.5	3.5	0.8	n/a
Oxtail Soup					
canned HEINZ	**37**	1.6	6.5	0.5	0.3
diluted CAMPBELL'S	**44**	1.4	5.1	1.9	n/a
Cup-A-Soup, per sachet					
BATCHELORS	**83**	2.2	11.2	3.3	0.8
Parsnip & Carrot Soup					
WEIGHT WATCHERS	**25**	0.5	5.3	0.2	0.9

All amounts per 100g/100ml unless otherwise stated	Cal kcal	Pro g	Carb g	Fat g	Fibre g
Pea & Ham Soup BAXTERS	**55**	3	8.3	1.1	1.2
Potato, Leek & Bacon Chilled Soup BAXTERS	**83**	2	6.1	5.6	0.7
Potato & Leek Soup BAXTERS	**45**	1.1	8.1	0.9	0.8
GRANNY'S	**38**	0.8	8.7	0.1	n/a
Rich Tomato & Basil Cup-A-Soup, per sachet BATCHELORS	**97**	1.3	17.3	2.5	1.3
Rich Woodland Mushroom Cup-A-Soup, per sachet BATCHELORS	**110**	1.3	15	5	2.3
Royal Game Soup BAXTERS	**41**	2.8	6.2	0.5	0.2
Scotch Broth					
BAXTERS	**47**	1.9	7.5	1	0.9
GRANNY'S	**55**	1.6	8.9	1.4	n/a
HEINZ	**35**	1.2	5.8	0.7	0.6
chilled BAXTERS	**39**	1.7	5.8	1	0.6
diluted CAMPBELL'S	**41**	1.1	5.4	1.8	n/a
Scotch Vegetable Soup BAXTERS	**43**	1.9	7.4	0.6	1.2
Scottish Pea & Bacon Soups of the World KNORR	**385**	18.4	53.5	10	4
Scottish Vegetable Soup with Lentils & Beef HEINZ	**52**	3.4	8.2	0.7	1.2
Seafood Chowder BAXTERS	**75**	3.3	5.4	4.5	0.4

All amounts per 100g/100ml unless otherwise stated	Cal kcal	Pro g	Carb g	Fat g	Fibre g
Smoked Bacon & Three Bean Soup BAXTERS	54	2.7	8.9	0.8	1.7
Spicy Lentil & Vegetable Soup BAXTERS	51	2.2	9	0.7	1.1
Spicy Parsnip Soup					
BAXTERS	51	1.1	6.1	2.5	1.5
as sold KNORR	443	5.7	56	21.7	4
special HEINZ	56	1.3	7.8	2.2	1.6
Spicy Tomato & Rice with Sweetcorn Soup BAXTERS	45	1.3	9.2	0.3	0.5
Split Pea & Lentil Soup WEIGHT WATCHERS	32	1.6	6	0.2	0.6
Spring Vegetable Soup					
HEINZ	31	0.8	6.2	0.4	0.7
99% fat free, diluted CAMPBELL'S	21	0.5	4.6	0.1	n/a
Stilton & White Port Soup BAXTERS	88	2.5	5.4	6.3	0.3
Swedish Cauliflower & Broccoli Soups of the World, as sold KNORR	425	7	41.8	25.5	3.9
Tangy Tomato Cup-A-Soup Extra, per sachet BATCHELORS	137	3.4	25.8	2.2	1.1
Thick Potato, Bacon & Onion Cup-A-Soup Extra, per sachet BATCHELORS	114	2.8	20.7	2.2	1.3

All amounts per 100g/100ml unless otherwise stated	Cal kcal	Pro g	Carb g	Fat g	Fibre g
Tomato Soup					
99% fat-free, diluted CAMPBELL'S	43	0.6	8	1	n/a
GRANNY'S	56	1.2	10.7	0.9	n/a
Cup-A-Soup, per sachet					
BATCHELORS	92	0.7	17.2	2.3	0.7
low calorie WEIGHT WATCHERS	25	0.7	4.6	0.5	0.3
with mascarpone cheese					
CARB OPTIONS	37	0.7	4.4	1.9	0.5
Tomato & Brown Lentil Soup					
BAXTERS	46	2.4	8.3	0.3	1.3
Tomato & Butter Bean Soup					
BAXTERS	53	1.9	8.6	1.2	1.8
Tomato & Lentil Soup HEINZ	54	2.7	10.4	0.2	1
Tomato & Red Pepper Soup					
99% fat-free, diluted CAMPBELL'S	41	0.5	7.5	1	n/a
as sold KNORR	403	7.7	50.7	18.7	5.3
Tomato & Vegetable Soup					
Cup-A-Soup, per sachet					
BATCHELORS	108	2.8	18.4	2.6	2.1
Vegetable Soup					
HEINZ	43	1	8.2	0.7	0.9
diluted CAMPBELL'S	38	0.8	6.7	0.8	n/a
Chunky BAXTERS	40	1.6	7.7	0.3	1.1
Country HEINZ	51	2.3	9.3	0.5	1.1
Country WEIGHT WATCHERS	30	1.1	5.9	0.2	1

All amounts per 100g/100ml unless otherwise stated	Cal kcal	Pro g	Carb g	Fat g	Fibre g
Hearty, 99% fat free, diluted					
CAMPBELL'S	**31**	0.8	6.1	0.4	n/a
sachet, as sold WEIGHT WATCHERS	**57**	1.2	10.4	1.2	0.5
Watercress Soup, as sold KNORR	**414**	11.1	51.1	18.5	1.7
Winter Vegetable Soup					
HEINZ	**46**	2.8	8.2	0.2	1.1
WEIGHT WATCHERS	**31**	1.6	6	0.1	0.8

SUGAR & SWEETENERS

All amounts per 100g/100ml unless otherwise stated	Cal kcal	Pro g	Carb g	Fat g	Fibre g
Amber Sugar Crystals					
TATE & LYLE	**398**	Tr	99.9	0	0
Date Syrup MERIDIAN FOODS LTD	**292**	1.2	71.5	0.1	Tr
Golden Syrup	**298**	0.3	79	0	0
TATE & LYLE	**325**	0.5	80.5	0	0
Icing Sugar TATE & LYLE	**398**	0	99.5	0	0
Jaggery	**367**	0.5	97.2	0	n/a
Maple Syrup, organic					
MERIDIAN FOODS LTD	**344**	Tr	85.3	0.3	Tr
Molasses					
MERIDIAN FOODS LTD	**234**	2.5	56.1	Tr	Tr
organic MERIDIAN FOODS LTD	**234**	2.5	56	Tr	Tr
Sugar					
caster TATE & LYLE	**400**	0	99.9	0	0
cube, white TATE & LYLE	**400**	0	99.9	0	0
dark brown, soft TATE & LYLE	**378**	0.4	94.5	0	0
Demerara, cane TATE & LYLE	**400**	Tr	99.2	0	Tr
granulated TATE & LYLE	**400**	0	99.9	0	0
light brown, soft TATE & LYLE	**384**	0.1	95.8	0	0
preserving TATE & LYLE	**400**	0	99.9	0	0
Treacle					
black	**257**	1.2	67.2	0	n/a
black LYLE'S	**290**	1.7	64	0	0

SWEETS & CHOCOLATE

All amounts per 100g/100ml unless otherwise stated	Cal kcal	Pro g	Carb g	Fat g	Fibre g
Aero Nestlé					
bubbles	**527**	4.8	61.5	29.1	0.4
caramel	**490**	5.5	60.6	25.1	0.6
Irish cream	**528**	5	61.9	28.9	0.4
milk chocolate	**518**	6.8	58.1	28.7	0.8
mint	**529**	5.5	61.4	29	0.4
sticky toffee	**528**	5	61.9	28.9	0.4
After Eight Mints Nestlé					
chocolate mint straws	**541**	4.9	54	33	5.3
dark chocolate	**417**	2.5	72.9	12.8	1.1
orange	**417**	2.5	72.6	12.9	1.1
white chocolate	**422**	2.6	76.9	11.6	n/a
American Hard Gums Trebor Bassett	**330**	0	82	0	0
Aniseed Imperials Trebor Bassett	**395**	0	98	0	n/a
Black Jack Chews Trebor Bassett	**400**	1	85	6	n/a
Black Jack Chew Bars Trebor Bassett	**400**	1	85	6	n/a
Blue Riband Nestlé	**513**	4.8	66.4	25.3	1.1
Bonbons					
fruit Trebor Bassett	**380**	0	94	0	n/a
lemon Trebor Bassett	**425**	0	84	10	n/a
strawberry Trebor Bassett	**380**	0	76	9	n/a
toffee Trebor Bassett	**420**	0	84	9	n/a

All amounts per 100g/100ml unless otherwise stated	Cal kcal	Pro g	Carb g	Fat g	Fibre g
Boost CADBURY					
glucose	**515**	6	57	30	n/a
guarana	**510**	6	58	29	n/a
Bounty MARS	**471**	3.7	56.4	25.6	5.2
Bournville CADBURY	**500**	4	61	26	n/a
Breakaway NESTLÉ					
Caramac	**519**	6.6	57.4	29.2	2
milk chocolate	**496**	6.8	59.7	25.5	2.5
Candy Sticks TREBOR BASSETT	**390**	1	90	3	n/a
Caramac NESTLÉ	**563**	5.8	54.4	35.8	0
Caramel CADBURY	**480**	5	62	24	n/a
Caramels TREBOR BASSETT	**480**	5	62	24	n/a
Grannymels ITONA	**456**	3.8	84.2	11.5	n/a
Chewing Gum WRIGLEY					
Airwaves blackcurrant	**155**	0	n/a	0	0
Airwaves cherry menthol	**150**	0	n/a	0	0
Airwaves Vapour Release	**155**	0	n/a	0	0
Doublemint	**306**	0	n/a	0	0
Extra Cool Breeze	**165**	0	N	0	0
Extra Ice	**155**	0	N	0	0
Extra Mountain Frost	**150**	0	N	0	0
Extra Peppermint	**155**	0	N	0	0
Extra Spearmint	**165**	0	N	0	0
Extra Thin Ice Strips	**125**	0	N	0	0

All amounts per 100g/100ml unless otherwise stated	Cal kcal	Pro g	Carb g	Fat g	Fibre g
Juicy Fruit	**295**	0	N	0	0
Juicy Fruit, strappleberry	**300**	0	N	0	0
Orbit, Ice White	**170**	0	N	0	0
Orbit, peppermint, xylitol	**175**	0	N	0	0
Orbit, Professional	**150**	0	N	0	0
Orbit, Professional White	**155**	0	N	0	0
Orbit, spearmint, xylitol	**175**	0	N	0	0
Spearmint	**281**	0	N	0	0
Chewits LEAF	**378**	0.3	86.9	2.7	0
extremely sour	**376**	0.3	84.9	2.6	0
Chocolate Cream, Fry's CADBURY	**415**	3	70	14	n/a
Chocolate Eclairs CADBURY	**455**	4	70	18	n/a
Chocolate Orange TERRY'S	**532**	7.4	57.8	29.5	2.1
Chocolate Truffles ELIZABETH SHAW					
with Cointreau	**474**	3.7	64.1	21.8	0.9
with Irish Cream	**474**	3.8	64.1	22.1	0.9
with Tia Maria	**474**	3.7	64	21.9	0.9
Chocolate					
milk	**520**	7.7	56.9	30.7	n/a
milk, organic GREEN & BLACK	**542**	9.5	54	32	n/a
plain	**510**	5	63.5	28	n/a
plain, organic GREEN & BLACK	**576**	7.5	45.5	40.5	n/a
white	**529**	8	58.3	30.9	n/a
white, organic GREEN & BLACK	**577**	7.5	52.5	37.5	n/a

All amounts per 100g/100ml unless otherwise stated	Cal kcal	Pro g	Carb g	Fat g	Fibre g
Chocolate, Maya Gold, organic					
GREEN & BLACK	552	6	56.5	33.5	n/a
Chomp CADBURY	460	3	68	20	n/a
Chunky CADBURY	515	5	59	29	n/a
Creme Egg CADBURY	445	3	71	16	n/a
Crunch NESTLÉ					
milk chocolate	513	6.7	59.7	27.5	1.5
white chocolate	519	7.5	60.5	27.6	n/a
Crunchie CADBURY	470	4	72	18	n/a
Crunchie Nuggets CADBURY	460	4	73	17	n/a
Curly Wurly CADBURY	450	4	69	18	n/a
Curly Wurly Squirlies CADBURY	450	4	69	18	n/a
Dairy Milk Chocolate CADBURY	525	8	56	30	n/a
Dairy Milk Tasters CADBURY	530	8	56	31	n/a
Double Decker CADBURY	465	5	65	21	n/a
Dream CADBURY	555	5	60	33	n/a
Drifter NESTLÉ	478	3.7	67.3	21.5	0.8
Energy Tablets LUCOZADE SPORT	361	Tr	89.2	0	n/a
lemon	360	0	88.8	0	n/a
orange	361	Tr	89.2	0	n/a

All amounts per 100g/100ml unless otherwise stated	Cal kcal	Pro g	Carb g	Fat g	Fibre g
Everton Mints TREBOR BASSETT	**390**	0	93	2	n/a
Flake CADBURY	**525**	8	55	31	n/a
Fruit & Nut Chocolate CADBURY	**490**	8	55	26	n/a
Fruit & Nut Tasters CADBURY	**510**	9	51	30	n/a
Fruit Gums TREBOR BASSETT	**335**	6	77	0	n/a
NESTLÉ	**342**	4.7	80.8	0.2	0
Fruit Pastilles NESTLÉ	**351**	4.4	83.7	0	0
Fruit Salad Chews TREBOR BASSETT	**400**	1	85	6	n/a
Fruit Salad Chew Bar TREBOR BASSETT	**400**	1	85	6	n/a
Fruitang TREBOR BASSETT	**400**	1	83	6	n/a
Fudge CADBURY	**435**	3	73	15	n/a
Fuse CADBURY	**485**	7	59	25	n/a
Galaxy chocolate MARS	**539**	6.8	56.9	31.6	1.5
fruit & hazelnut	**528**	6.5	54.7	31.4	n/a
hazelnut	**582**	7.8	49.4	39.2	n/a
Galaxy Promises MARS					
Caramel Crunch	**540**	6.1	57.5	31.8	n/a
Cocoa Crisp	**533**	5.6	55.8	32	n/a
Rich Coffee	**535**	5.7	54.4	32.8	n/a
Roast Hazelnut	**544**	6.4	55.6	32.9	n/a
Just Fruit Jellies TREBOR BASSETT	**380**	0	94	0	n/a

All amounts per 100g/100ml unless otherwise stated	Cal kcal	Pro g	Carb g	Fat g	Fibre g
Kit Kat NESTLÉ					
4-finger dark chocolate	**500**	6	59.2	27	1.9
4-finger milk chocolate	**508**	6	61.5	26.4	1.1
4-finger white chocolate	**524**	801	60.4	27.8	0.6
Chunky milk chocolate	**518**	5.4	60.8	28.1	1
Chunky white chocolate	**525**	8	58.3	28.9	0.4
low carb	**438**	9.2	28.3	8.9	1.3
orange	**496**	4.6	69.3	23	0.8
Liaison GALAXY	**500**	6.8	52.9	34.6	n/a
Lion Bar NESTLÉ	**489**	4.7	67.6	22.2	0.8
peanut	**522**	7.1	56.9	29.6	n/a
Liquorice Allsorts TREBOR BASSETT	**350**	2	76	5	n/a
Lockets MARS	**383**	0	95.8	0	n/a
M & Ms MARS					
chocolate	**490**	5.1	69.4	21.4	2.8
crispy shell	**510**	5.3	64.3	25.7	2.7
peanut	**520**	10.3	58.4	27.2	2.1
Maltesers MARS	**484**	8.7	58.6	23.8	1.1
Marble CADBURY	**530**	9	54	31	n/a
Mars Bar MARS	**449**	4.2	69	17.4	1.2
Matchmakers NESTLÉ					
Coolmint	**477**	4.3	69.7	20.1	0.9
White	**505**	5.7	67.6	23.5	0
Zingy Orange	**475**	4.4	69.5	20	0.9

All amounts per 100g/100ml unless otherwise stated	Cal kcal	Pro g	Carb g	Fat g	Fibre g
Minstrels GALAXY	506	5.3	71	22.3	n/a
Milk Tray CADBURY	490	5	61	26	n/a
Milky Way MARS	440	3.4	74.8	14.1	1.7
Mint Creams TREBOR BASSETT	365	0	92	0	n/a
Mint Crisp CADBURY	485	6	64	23	n/a
Mint Crisps ELIZABETH SHAW					
Coffee	473	2.9	66	21.3	5.3
Dark	473	2.8	74	21.4	4.5
Milk & Dark	485	3.4	65.6	23.2	3.9
Milk Chocolate	499	4.2	68.8	21.4	1
Orange	470	2.8	66.9	21.2	4.5
Mint Imperials TREBOR BASSETT	395	0	98	0	n/a
Mintetts G. PAYNE & CO	395	Tr	92.7	27	n/a
Munchies NESTLÉ	487	5	63.1	23.8	0.5
Mint	432	3.8	67.5	16.4	1.6
Murray Mints TREBOR BASSETT	410	0	90	5.3	n/a
Nougat TREBOR BASSETT	375	4	82	4	n/a
Nuts about Caramel CADBURY	485	5	58	26	n/a
Orange Cream, Fry's CADBURY	420	3	72	14	n/a
Pear Drops TREBOR BASSETT	390	0	96	0	n/a
Peppermints	393	0.5	102.7	0.7	n/a

All amounts per 100g/100ml unless otherwise stated	Cal kcal	Pro g	Carb g	Fat g	Fibre g
Peppermint Cream, Fry's CADBURY	425	3	73	14	n/a
Picnic CADBURY	470	7	59	23	n/a
Polo Fruits NESTLÉ	385	0	95.1	0	0
berrylicious	238	0	98.7	0	0
citrus sharp	394	0	96.8	1	0
Polo Mints NESTLÉ	402	0	98.2	1	0
spearmint	401	0	98.1	1	0
sugar-free	238	0	99.1	0	0
Polo Smoothies NESTLÉ					
blackcurrant	412	0.1	88.4	6.8	0
clear ice	386	0	96.4	0	0
spearmint clear	386	0	96.9	0	0
strawberry	412	0.1	88.4	6.8	0
sunshine fruits	412	0.1	88.4	6.8	0
Poppets G. PAYNE & CO					
peanut	544	16.4	37	37	n/a
peanut & raisin	460	10	53	24.5	n/a
raisins	409	4.8	66	14	n/a
white chocolate & raisins	286	5.9	63.6	16.6	n/a
Refreshers TREBOR BASSETT	375	0	90	0	n/a
cola	375	0	90	0	n/a
gums	335	4	78	0	n/a
lollies	375	0	92	0	n/a
Revels MARS	476	5	65.8	20.9	n/a

All amounts per 100g/100ml unless otherwise stated	Cal kcal	Pro g	Carb g	Fat g	Fibre g
Ripple GALAXY	**528**	6.9	59.3	29.3	n/a
Rolo NESTLÉ	**471**	3.2	68.5	20.5	0.3
low carb	**346**	6.4	10.3	26.3	0.4
Roses Assortment CADBURY	**495**	5	61	26	n/a
Schnapps Shots, all flavours ELIZABETH SHAW	**481**	3.7	62.2	22	0.9
Sherbet Fountain TREBOR BASSETT	**345**	1	83	0	n/a
Skittles MARS	**404**	0	91.5	4.2	0
Snack CADBURY					
Sandwich Chocolate	**515**	7	61	27	n/a
Shortcake	**520**	7	63	27	n/a
Wafer	**525**	6	61	29	n/a
Snickers, each MARS	**280**	4	35	14	1
Snowbites CADBURY	**550**	4	60	33	n/a
Softfruits TREBOR BASSETT	**380**	0	95	0	n/a
Softmints TREBOR BASSETT	**374**	0.1	88	2.3	0
mini	**350**	1	81	3	n/a
peppermint	**380**	0	95	0	n/a
spearmint	**375**	0	94	0	n/a
Spearmint Imperials TREBOR BASSETT	**395**	0	98	0	n/a
Spira CADBURY	**525**	8	56	30	n/a

All amounts per 100g/100ml unless otherwise stated	Cal kcal	Pro g	Carb g	Fat g	Fibre g
Starbar CADBURY	**540**	9.1	55	31.6	n/a
Starburst MARS	**411**	0.3	85.3	7.6	n/a
Sourburst	**307**	4.2	72.6	0	n/a
Sweets, boiled	**327**	Tr	87.1	Tr	n/a
Tequila Shots, all flavours					
ELIZABETH SHAW	**481**	3.7	62.2	22	0.9
Timeout CADBURY	**530**	6	58	31	n/a
Toblerone TERRY'S	**530**	5.4	58	30.5	2.6
Toffees, mixed	**426**	2.2	66.7	18.6	n/a
Grannymels Mint ITONA	**465**	3.8	84.2	1.5	n/a
Toffee Crisp NESTLÉ	**511**	4.3	60.6	27.9	0.8
Toffo NESTLÉ	**452**	2.1	70.1	18.1	0
Topic MARS	**502**	6.3	60.3	26.2	1.6
Trebor Extra Strong Mints					
TREBOR BASSETT	**395**	0	98	0	n/a
extra strong menthol & eucalyptus	**385**	0	99	0	n/a
extra strong spearmint	**395**	0	99	0	n/a
Trebor Mints TREBOR BASSETT	**395**	1	97	0	n/a
Tunes MARS	**392**	0	98.1	0	n/a
Turkish Delight Fry's CADBURY	**365**	2	73	7	n/a

All amounts per 100g/100ml unless otherwise stated	Cal kcal	Pro g	Carb g	Fat g	Fibre g
Selfline TREBOR BASSETT	**435**	4	64	18	n/a
without nuts	**295**	0.6	77.9	0	n/a
Twirl CADBURY	**525**	7	56	31	n/a
Twix MARS	**493**	4.7	63.7	24.4	1.6
Twixels MARS	**514**	4.9	64.2	26.4	n/a
Viscount Mint BURTON'S	**522**	5.1	60.6	28.8	1.3
Vodka Shots, all flavours ELIZABETH SHAW	**481**	3.7	61.9	22	0.9
Walnut Whip, vanilla NESTLÉ	**495**	5.9	60.8	25.4	0.6
Wholenut Chocolate CADBURY	**545**	9	48	35	n/a
Wholenut Tasters CADBURY	**565**	10	44	39	n/a
Wine Gums MAYNARD'S	**330**	6	76.7	Tr	n/a
Wispa CADBURY	**550**	6	55	34	n/a
Yorkie NESTLÉ					
biscuit	**510**	6.7	60.4	26.8	1.3
milk chocolate	**537**	6.1	57.3	31.5	0.7
raisin & biscuit	**487**	5.9	60.5	24.6	n/a

VEGETARIAN

All amounts per 100g/100ml unless otherwise stated	Cal kcal	Pro g	Carb g	Fat g	Fibre g
Baked Beans & Vegetable Sausages HEINZ	105	6	12.2	3.6	2.9
Bolognese Beanfeast, as served BATCHELORS	62	5.2	8.1	1	2.1
Burgers, flame-grilled LINDA MCCARTNEY FOODS	174	17.9	13.8	5.2	3.3
Cauliflower Cheese BIRDS EYE	93	4.8	6	5.5	1.2
Chargrilled Vegetable Sauce, as sold BERTOLLI	53	2	6.9	2	1.3
Deep Country Pies LINDA MCCARTNEY FOODS	243	6.2	65	13.1	1.1
Gravy Granules for Vegetable Dishes, as sold OXO	309	8.4	59.3	4.2	3.1
Italian Tomato Pasta Sauces GO ORGANIC					
and aubergine	67	1.2	3.9	5.2	1
and black olive	68	1.1	3.6	5.5	0.9
and red chilli	75	1.3	5	5.5	1.2
and sweet basil	64	1.2	4.3	4.7	0.9
and sweet pepper	77	1.3	5.8	5.4	1.2
Macaroni Cheese, each BIRDS EYE	470	17	67	15	2.4
frozen ROSS	109	4.2	16.2	3.1	1.3
Pasta Presto, each FINDUS	150	5.5	16	7	n/a
Mediterranean Vegetable Sauce, as sold BERTOLLI	88	1.7	4.1	7.2	0.7

All amounts per 100g/100ml unless otherwise stated	Cal kcal	Pro g	Carb g	Fat g	Fibre g
Mushroom, Garlic, Oregano & Tomato Sauce, as sold BERTOLLI	**90**	1.9	3.8	7.5	0.9
Onions & Garlic Sauce RAGU	**37**	1.4	7.7	0.1	0.9
OY PROVAMEL					
banana flavour soya milk	**79**	3.8	10.7	2.2	0.6
chocolate flavour soya milk	**75**	3.8	9.8	2.2	1.1
strawberry flavour soya milk	**68**	3.8	8	2.2	0.6
Pâté					
Herb & Garlic TARTEX	**218**	7	7	18	n/a
Herb Provençal GRANOVITA	**240**	4	4	5.8	n/a
Original GRANOVITA	**240**	10.7	2.5	18.8	n/a
Mushroom TARTEX	**214**	7	6	18	n/a
Yeast TARTEX	**214**	7	6	18	n/a
Spicy Mexican GRANOVITA	**216**	6	3	20	n/a
Wild Mushroom GRANOVITA	**222**	10	5	18	n/a
Quorn, myco-protein	**92**	14.1	1.9	3.2	N
Ravioli in Tomato Sauce HEINZ	**73**	3.1	13.2	0.8	0.3
Rice Drink PROVAMEL					
calcium enriched	**50**	0.1	9.6	1.2	0
organic	**49**	0.1	9.5	1.2	0
Roast Vegetable Flavour Gravy Granules, as sold BISTO	**317**	2.1	64.2	5.7	1.1
Sausage Rolls LINDA MCCARTNEY FOODS	**273**	9.7	28.2	13.5	2.5
Sausages LINDA MCCARTNEY FOODS	**252**	23.2	8.6	13.8	1.2

All amounts per 100g/100ml unless otherwise stated	Cal kcal	Pro g	Carb g	Fat g	Fibre g
Shepherd's Pie LINDA MCCARTNEY FOODS	**84**	3.7	12.3	2.2	2.3
Sorbet					
fruit	**97**	0.2	24.8	0.3	1
lemon	**128**	0	32	0	0
Soya Bean Curd: *see* **Tofu**					
Soya Chunks HOLLAND & BARRETT					
flavoured	**345**	50	35	1	4
natural	**345**	50	35	1	4
Soya Curd: *see* **Tofu**					
Soya Dream PROVAMEL	**178**	3	1.7	17.7	1.1
Soya Flour					
full fat	**447**	36.8	23.5	23.5	n/a
low fat	**352**	45.3	28.2	7.2	n/a
Soya Milk					
chocolate, organic PROVAMEL	**81**	3.8	10.7	2.4	1.2
sweetened	**43**	3.1	2.5	2.4	Tr
sweetened, organic PROVAMEL	**46**	3.7	2.8	2.2	0.6
unsweetened	**26**	2.4	0.5	1.6	0.5
unsweetened HOLLAND & BARRETT	**35**	3.7	0.1	2.2	0.6
vanilla flavoured, organic PROVAMEL	**61**	3.8	6.5	2.1	0.3
Soya Mince HOLLAND & BARRETT					
flavoured	**345**	50	35	1	4
unflavoured	**345**	50	35	1	4

All amounts per 100g/100ml unless otherwise stated	Cal kcal	Pro g	Carb g	Fat g	Fibre g
Sweet Chilli, Red Onion & Tomato Sauce, as sold BERTOLLI	91	1.7	4.9	7.2	0.7
Sweet Pepper & Tomato Sauce, as sold BERTOLLI	89	1.5	4.3	7.2	0.5
Thai Curry Sauces, as sold GO ORGANIC					
mild Thai curry with lime & coconut	125	1.6	6.2	10.4	1.2
Thai green curry with coriander & lime	124	1.6	6.3	10.3	1.3
Thai red curry with galangal & red chili	99	1.6	5.5	7.8	1.3
Tofu (soya bean curd)					
steamed	73	8.1	0.7	4.2	n/a
steamed, fried	261	23.5	2	17.7	n/a
Tomato, Red Wine & Shallots Sauce, as sold BERTOLLI	49	2	6.1	1.9	1.2
Tomato, Roasted Garlic & Mushrooms Sauce, as sold BERTOLLI	47	1.9	5.3	1.9	1.2
Tomato, Romano & Garlic Sauce, as sold BERTOLLI	66	2.5	7.2	3.1	1.2
Vegemite KRAFT	191	25.6	19.5	0.9	0
Vegetable Casserole, frozen ROSS	96	3.4	15.4	2.3	2

All amounts per 100g/100ml unless otherwise stated	Cal kcal	Pro g	Carb g	Fat g	Fibre g
Vegetable Granulated Stock					
KNORR	**199**	8.5	39.9	0.6	0.9
Vegetable Stock VECON	**171**	25	17.5	1.5	3.5
Vegetable Stock Cubes,					
prepared KNORR	**10**	0.3	0.3	0.9	Tr
as sold OXO	**258**	9.8	45.3	4.2	1.7
Vegetable Tikka Masala Curry					
Break PATAK	**112**	2.4	13.6	5.4	n/a
Vegetarian Double Gloucester					
Cheese HOLLAND & BARRETT	**405**	24.6	0.1	34	0
Vegetarian Mild Cheddar Cheese					
HOLLAND & BARRETT	**412**	25.5	0.1	34.4	0
Vegetarian Red Leicester Cheese					
HOLLAND & BARRETT	**401**	24.3	0.1	33.7	0
Vegetarian Tandoori Vegetable					
Pasty HOLLAND & BARRETT	**188**	4.4	29.9	5.7	1.8
Yofu, organic, each PROVAMEL					
peach & mango	**128**	4.8	20.5	2.8	1.5
red cherry	**125**	4.8	20.1	2.8	1.5
strawberry	**135**	4.8	19.5	4	0.3

FAST FOOD

All amounts per 100g/100ml unless otherwise stated	Cal kcal	Pro g	Carb g	Fat g	Fibre g
McDONALD'S					
Apple Pie, each	**230**	2.2	26.5	12.8	1.1
Big Breakfast, each	**591**	26.2	39.8	36.3	4
Big Mac, each	**493**	26.7	44	22.9	5.9
Cheeseburger, each	**318**	17	34.6	12.7	1.9
double	**438**	26.6	33.3	22.1	3.1
Chicken Caesar Flatbread, per portion	**328**	23.5	46.4	5.4	1.8
Chicken Caesar Salad, per portion					
Crispy Chicken with dressing & croutons	**451**	33.1	31	22.3	4.9
Crispy Chicken without dressing & croutons	**337**	28.6	15.6	18.4	3.7
Grilled Chicken with dressing & croutons	**354**	31.6	28.7	12.8	4
Chicken Grill	**76**	10.9	5.4	1.3	0.1
Chicken McNuggets (6)	**208**	14.2	7.9	13.3	1
Chicken Ranch Salad, per portion					
Crispy Chicken with dressing	**451**	34.1	26.2	23.9	3.7
Crispy Chicken without dressing	**382**	31.4	16.1	21.9	3.7
Grilled Chicken with dressing	**361**	33.3	23.9	15	2.8
Grilled Chicken without dressing	**292**	30.6	13.8	13	2.8
Egg McMuffin	**281**	15.5	25.9	12.3	2.5

All amounts per 100g/100ml unless otherwise stated	Cal kcal	Pro g	Carb g	Fat g	Fibre g
Filet-O-Fish, each	**385**	15.9	40.4	17.8	2
French Fries, small, per portion	**206**	2.9	28.3	9	2.8
Fruit & Yogurt, per portion	**150**	4	22.8	2.9	1.6
Fruit Bag, per portion	**43**	0.2	10.4	0.1	1.8
Grilled Chicken Pasta Salad, per portion					
with dressing	**433**	29.2	50.3	14.1	4.5
without dressing	**420**	28.9	47.6	12.9	4.2
Hamburger, each	**271**	14.3	33.8	8.8	1.9
Hash Browns	**138**	1.4	15.8	7.7	1.7
McBacon Roll	**349**	16.5	37.3	14	2.1
McChicken Premiere, each	**481**	24.5	50.1	19.9	3.9
McChicken Sandwich, each	**375**	16.5	38.6	17.2	3.8
Milkshake, vanilla, small, each	**383**	10.8	62.7	10.1	0
Orange Juice, bottle	**123**	0	29.3	0	Tr
Pancakes & Syrup	**532**	5.1	873.7	15.9	1.2
Quarter Pounder with cheese	**516**	31.2	37.5	26.7	3.7

WIMPY

All day breakfast	**715**	30.3	46	49.5	3.7
Bacon & egg in a bun	**345**	18.8	32.3	15.4	1.7

All amounts per 100g/100ml unless otherwise stated	Cal kcal	Pro g	Carb g	Fat g	Fibre g
Bacon Cheeseburger	**345**	19.1	32.3	15.3	1.7
Bacon Classic Cheeseburger	**415**	25	33.3	20.2	2.4
Bacon in a bun	**230**	10.3	32.3	6.7	1.7
BBQ Pork Rib in a Bun	**555**	30.2	67.9	19.4	3.6
Bender, egg & chips	**656**	25.8	46.6	41	4
Cheeseburger	**315**	16.7	32.3	13.1	1.7
Chicken chunks & chips	**770**	27.4	79.9	38	4.2
Chicken in a bun	**435**	16.3	42	22.2	1.9
Chips	**295**	3.7	42.4	12.1	3.5
Classic Kingsize	**550**	26.2	33.3	30.3	2.4
Fish in a bun	**615**	34.4	64	13.5	3.6
Fish 'n' Chips	**490**	27.8	47.4	21.2	4.2
Hamburger	**270**	13.7	32.3	9.6	1.7
Hot 'n' Spicy Chicken in a bun	**430**	18.5	45.8	19.7	2.4
Quarterpounder	**540**	28.2	42.3	29.9	6.7
with cheese	**585**	31.1	42.3	33.4	6.7
Spicy Beanburger	**520**	16.1	68.7	22	16.9
Toasted Tea Cake & butter	**245**	58	35.2	9.8	1.7
Wimpy Classic	**340**	19.6	33.3	14.5	2.4
with cheese	**385**	22.6	33.3	18	2.4

All amounts per 100g/100ml unless otherwise stated	Cal kcal	Pro g	Carb g	Fat g	Fibre g
Wimpy Classic Grill	**820**	39.3	46.2	53.5	3.7
bacon grill	**740**	36.7	46.4	49.1	3.9
quarterpounder grill	**955**	50.6	46.4	63.5	3.9
Wimpy Double Decker	**525**	51.2	42.3	51.4	6.7

BURGER KING

Cheeseburger	**350**	19	31	150	1
Chicken Caesar Salad	**190**	25	9	7	1
Chicken Whopper	**570**	38	48	25	4
Croissan'wich, with egg & cheese	**300**	12	26	17	Tr
French Fries, Small	**230**	3	29	11	2
Hamburger	**310**	17	30	13	1
Onion Rings, Medium	**320**	4	40	16	3
Veggie Burger	**420**	23	46	16	7
Whopper	**700**	31	52	42	4

PIZZA HUT

BBQ Chicken Wings, portion	**412**	38.6	8.3	24.7	n/a
BBQ Dip, portion	**39**	0.4	9.4	0.1	n/a
Caesar Salad, portion	**344**	11.7	28.8	20.2	n/a

All amounts per 100g/100ml unless otherwise stated	Cal kcal	Pro g	Carb g	Fat g	Fibre g
Chicken Caesar Salad, portion	**459**	46.1	21.2	21.2	n/a
Dippin' Chicken, portion	**330**	24.2	26.3	14.3	n/a
Garlic Bread, portion	**407**	10.1	55.4	16.1	n/a
Garlic Bread with Cheese, portion	**587**	31.3	43.2	32.2	n/a
Garlic Mushrooms, crispy coated, portion	**240**	5.5	31.6	10.1	n/a
Hawaiian Medium Pan, per slice	**245**	12.2	25.8	10.3	n/a
Hi-Light, Medium, per slice					
Chicken	**189**	10.8	23.9	5.5	n/a
Ham	**184**	9.9	23.8	5.5	n/a
Vegetarian	**170**	7.9	23	5.1	n/a
Lasagne, portion	**656**	30.4	56.3	33.4	n/a
Margherita Medium Pan, per slice	**301**	15.4	26.3	15	n/a
Meat Feast Medium Pan, per slice	**337**	17.6	26.6	17.7	n/a
Nachos, portion	**434**	15.7	42.3	22.4	n/a
Potato Skins, portion	**571**	36.2	32	34.2	n/a
Potato Wedges, portion	**328**	4.7	46.4	13.8	n/a
Sour Cream & Chive dip, portion	**51**	0.1	12.2	0.1	n/a

All amounts per 100g/100ml unless otherwise stated	Cal kcal	Pro g	Carb g	Fat g	Fibre g
Stuffed Crust, per slice					
Margherita	**338**	18.1	39.8	11.8	n/a
Meat Feast	**417**	24.5	39.1	18.1	n/a
Vegetable Supreme	**320**	16.9	39.7	10.5	n/a
Supreme Medium Pan, per slice	**309**	14.5	28.3	15.3	n/a
Sweet Chilli Sauce, portion	**51**	0.1	12.2	0.1	n/a
Tagliatelle Carbonara, portion	**908**	27.2	83.5	51.7	n/a
The Edge, per slice					
Meaty	**110**	6.1	7.3	5.7	n/a
The Veggie	**87**	4.3	8.5	3.4	n/a
The Works	**104**	5.6	8.6	4.6	n/a
The Italian Medium, per slice					
Margherita	**269**	11.6	32.9	10.1	n/a
Meat Feast	**301**	12.8	33.1	13.1	n/a
Vegetable Supreme	**236**	10.6	30.7	7.9	n/a
Vegetarian Supreme Medium Pan, per slice	**266**	12.1	27.3	12.1	n/a
Warm Chicken Salad, portion	**244**	30.9	19.6	4.5	n/a

DOMINO'S PIZZA

BBQ Dip, per portion	**46**	0.3	11.2	0	0
Cheese & Tomato, medium, per slice	**136**	7.1	20.7	2.7	1.7

All amounts per 100g/100ml unless otherwise stated	Cal kcal	Pro g	Carb g	Fat g	Fibre g
Chicken Dunkers, per portion	55	4.1	4.3	2.4	0.2
Chicken Strippers, per portion	64	4.8	3	3.7	0.2
Coleslaw, per portion	254	2.2	12.6	21.4	n/a
Deluxe, medium, per slice	178	9.9	20.3	6.4	1.7
Full House, medium, per slice	197	11.1	20.3	7.2	1.3
Garlic Pizza Bread, per slice	145	8.8	16.2	5	1.5
Mighty Meaty, medium, per slice	192	12.2	20.9	6.6	1.6
Mixed Grill, medium, per slice	203	11.7	22.2	7.4	1.2
Pepperoni Passion, medium, per slice	198	12.9	21.4	9.1	2.1
Potato Wedges, per portion	316	4.5	49.3	11.2	5.6
Tandoori Hot, medium, per slice	154	10	21	3.3	1.4
Vegetarian Supreme, medium, per slice	138	8.5	21	2.3	1.7

PIZZA EXPRESS

American	753	35.3	87.3	32.4	n/a
American Hot	758	35.9	87.4	32.6	n/a
Cannelloni, per portion	556	20.9	38.7	35.4	n/a
Fiorentina	740	38.22	88.4	27.5	n/a

All amounts per 100g/100ml unless otherwise stated	Cal kcal	Pro g	Carb g	Fat g	Fibre g
La Reine	**665**	34.9	87.4	22.8	n/a
Lasagne Pasticciate, per portion	**579**	26.4	29.9	39.5	n/a
Margherita	**621**	29.3	87.3	20.4	n/a
Mushroom	**627**	30.1	87.5	20.6	n/a
Pollo, per portion	**573**	41.1	32.5	31.8	n/a
Quattro Formaggi	**636**	29.4	87.2	22.1	n/a
Salade Nicoise, per portion	**729**	40	65	37	n/a
Sloppy Giuseppe	**783**	41	97	33	n/a
Tortellini, per portion	**1116**	26.9	91.9	71.3	n/a

FISH & CHIPS

Chips, fried in oil	**239**	3.2	30.5	12.4	n/a
Cod, in batter, fried	**247**	16.1	11.7	15.4	n/a
Plaice, in batter, fried	**257**	15.2	12	16.8	n/a
Rock Salmon/Dogfish, in batter, fried	**295**	14.7	10.3	21.9	n/a
Skate, in batter, fried	**168**	14.7	4.9	10.1	n/a

BOOTS SHAPERS

Apple, Strawberry & Kiwi Fruit with Yogurt	**46**	4	3.8	1.6	1.7

All amounts per 100g/100ml unless otherwise stated	Cal kcal	Pro g	Carb g	Fat g	Fibre g
Bacon Bites, per pack	**93**	1.8	13	3.8	0.5
Blackcurrant & Blackberry Drink, per pack	**4**	Tr	Tr	Tr	Tr
BLT	**161**	9.3	23	3.4	3
Caramel Rice Snacks, per pack	**95**	1.6	21	0.5	0.1
Chargrilled Chicken Crisps	**482**	6.6	60	24	4
Cheddar & Red Onion Crisps, per pack	**96**	1.7	13	4.3	1.5
Cheese & Celery Sandwiches, per pack	**287**	20	42	4.1	5.4
Cheese & Onion Crinkle Crisps	**482**	6.6	60	24	4
Cheese & Tomato Sandwiches, per pack	**288**	20	42	4.6	4.4
Cheese Crackers, Mini, per pack	**97**	2.2	15	3.2	1.1
Cheese Curls, per pack	**68**	0.6	8	3.8	0.2
Cheese Puffs, per pack	**80**	1.1	10	3.8	0.1
Cheese Salad Hearty Roll, per pack	**306**	24	43	4.6	4.6
Chicken & Tomato Pasta, per pack	**318**	17	48	6.3	6.4
Chicken, Bacon & Tomato Sandwiches, per pack	**317**	23	41	6.9	3.5

All amounts per 100g/100ml unless otherwise stated	Cal kcal	Pro g	Carb g	Fat g	Fibre g
Chicken Caesar Salad, per pack	164	16	13	5.4	3.9
Chicken Fajita Salad, per pack	181	18	19	3.5	6.9
Chicken Fajita Wrap, per pack	327	22	48	5.6	3.7
Chicken Herb Salad Hearty Roll, per pack	266	21	38	3.4	3.9
Chicken Salad Baguette, per pack	230	13	34	4.8	2.9
Chicken Salad Sandwiches, per pack	317	26	40	5.9	8.8
Chicken Triple Sandwiches, per pack	434	33	58	7.7	5.2
Chocolate & Raisin Cereal Bar, per pack	94	1.1	21	2.1	0.7
Cloudy Lemonade, per pack	7	Tr	0.5	Tr	Tr
Cranberry Juice Drink, per pack	40	Tr	9.6	Tr	Tr
Cranberry, Raisin & Nut Cereal Bar, per pack	140	2.5	23	4.4	1.3
Crayfish & Rocket Sandwiches, per pack	291	19	45	3.8	4.3
Crispy Caramel Bar	345	3.4	76	12	0.4
Crunchy Apple Wedges	51	0.3	12	0.1	1.8
Crunchy Apple Wedges & Juicy Grapes	58	0.3	14	0.1	1.4

All amounts per 100g/100ml unless otherwise stated	Cal kcal	Pro g	Carb g	Fat g	Fibre g
Crunchy Cheese & Onion Rings,					
per pack	**56**	0.9	12	0.4	0.3
Dairy Smoothies, per pack					
Mango & banana	**149**	4.8	30	1.1	1
Probiotic banana	**148**	4	30	1.3	2.5
Strawberry	**136**	5.6	25	1.2	1.2
Double Chocolate Bar, per pack	**93**	0.8	17	2.3	0.2
Dried Apricots, per pack	**83**	2	18	0.3	3.2
Dried Fruit Medley, per pack	**139**	1	33	0.2	2.7
Dried Prunes, per pack	**75**	1.3	17	0.2	2.9
Egg Mayonnaise Sandwiches,					
per pack	**323**	23	47	4.8	3.7
Flatbread					
BBQ chicken	**159**	11	24	2.3	2
chicken fajita	**150**	11	21	2.6	1.8
chicken tikka	**164**	11	24	2.5	0.7
Italian chicken	**154**	9.4	19	4.4	1.9
Mexican bean	**153**	8	24	2.7	1.9
Mozzarella, tomato & basil	**178**	9.9	25	4.3	1.9
Fruit Salad					
Classic	**35**	0.7	7.9	0.1	1.3
Classic, large	**46**	0.6	11	0.1	1.5
Tropical	**39**	0.7	8.4	0.2	1.5
Tropical, large	**35**	0.6	7.5	0.3	0.8

All amounts per 100g/100ml unless otherwise stated	Cal kcal	Pro g	Carb g	Fat g	Fibre g
Fruit Selection Pack, per pack	85	1.2	20	0.2	2.6
Fruit Smoothies, 100%, per pack					
Citrus blend	120	1.8	28	Tr	0.8
Cranberry & blackcurrant	148	1	35	0.5	2
Raspberry & boysenberry	109	1.8	25	Tr	4
Strawberry & raspberry	123	0.8	29	0.5	1.5
Ham Salad Sandwiches, per pack	269	18	43	2.7	3.5
Honey & Mustard & Chicken Pasta Salad, per pack	341	20	51	6.4	5.3
Houmous & Fire Roasted Vegetable Salad, per pack	235	12	34	5.5	11
Jumbo Raisins & Sultanas, per pack	145	1.2	35	0.2	1
Lemon & Lime Drink, still, per pack	5	Tr	Tr	Tr	Tr
Melon & Grape	33	0.6	7.5	0.1	0.8
Milk Chocolate Orange Bitesize Roll, per pack	61	0.7	9	2.5	0.1
Mint Bar, per pack	83	0.6	16	3.2	0.3
Mint Bar Tubs, Mini, per pack	45	0.3	8.8	1.7	0.1
New York Style Salted Pretzels Mini, per pack	95	2.5	20	0.5	1.1

All amounts per 100g/100ml unless otherwise stated	Cal kcal	Pro g	Carb g	Fat g	Fibre g
Orange & Tangerine Drink, sparkling, per pack	8	Tr	0.7	Tr	Tr
Orange Drink, vitamin enriched, per pack	35	Tr	8	Tr	Tr
Orange Juice, per pack	123	2	28	0.3	0.8
Oriental Chicken Triple Sandwiches, per pack	421	33	59	5.7	7.4
Peach & Apricot Drink, per pack	5	Tr	Tr	Tr	Tr
Pineapple Chunks, Golden	44	0.4	10	0.2	1.2
Prawn Mayonnaise Sandwiches, per pack	287	19	42	4.6	5
Prawn Salad, per pack	120	11	5.4	5.9	1.6
Prawn Shells	493	6.4	65	23	0.9
Raspberry & Apple Drink, sparkling, per pack	9	Tr	0.2	Tr	Tr
Roast Chicken Sandwiches, per pack	297	28	32	66	6.5
Salmon & Cucumber Sandwiches, per pack	272	18	34	6.8	5.2
Salt & Pepper Kettle Crisps, per pack	89	1.4	11	4.4	1

All amounts per 100g/100ml unless otherwise stated	Cal kcal	Pro g	Carb g	Fat g	Fibre g
Salt & Vinegar Crinkle Crisps, per pack	**96**	1.3	12	4.8	0.8
Salt & Vinegar Crunchy Sticks, per pack	**96**	1.2	14	3.8	0.5
Salt & Vinegar Rice Snacks, per pack	**95**	1.8	19	1.4	0.9
Salt & Vinegar Spirals, per pack	**71**	0.5	10	3.5	0.3
Salted Tubes, per pack	**68**	0.8	9.3	3	0.5
Sea Salt & Black Pepper Crisps, per pack	**96**	1.3	12	4.8	0.8
Smokey Bacon Crinkle Crisps, per pack	**96**	1.3	12	4.8	0.5
Sour Cream & Chives Crisps	**96**	1.3	12	4.8	0.8
Stem Ginger Mini Cookies, per pack	**131**	1.7	23	3.5	0.6
Strawberry & Vanilla Drink, sparkling, per pack	**5**	Tr	Tr	Tr	Tr
Strawberry & Yogurt Cereal Bar, per pack	**87**	0.9	16	2.3	0.8
Strawberry Bar, per pack	**84**	2.5	79	12	0.2
Strawberry Bar Tubs, Mini, per pack	**43**	0.3	8.4	1.7	0.1

All amounts per 100g/100ml unless otherwise stated	Cal kcal	Pro g	Carb g	Fat g	Fibre g
Sweet Grapes	**64**	0.4	15	0.1	0.7
Sweet Thai Chilli Handcooked Crisps, per pack	**95**	1.5	13	4.2	1.5
Tomato & Basil Salad, per pack	**263**	18	37	5.1	6.1
Tomato & Mozzarella Salad, per pack	**287**	13	40	8.3	5.1
Tuna & Cucumber Sandwiches, per pack	**307**	24	41	5.3	3.5
Tuna & Sweetcorn Sandwiches, per pack	**323**	23	47	4	3.7
Tuna Crunch Baguette, per pack	**228**	14	35	3.5	3.1
Tuna Crunch Pasta, per pack	**323**	16	51	6.3	4.8
Tuna Nicoise Salad, per pack	**129**	18	6.3	3.8	4.6
Tuna Salad Hearty Roll, per pack	**263**	21	39	2.7	4.4
Turkey, Cranberry & Stuffing Sandwiches, per pack	**283**	25	37	4	5.6
Turkish Delight, per pack	**88**	0.5	23	2.4	0.5
Wraps					
Cheese & Bean Wrap	**166**	6.6	27	3.4	2.1
Chicken Salad	**152**	9.4	22	3.1	1.7
Sweet Chilli Chicken Wrap	**176**	12	27	2.2	2

KIDS' FOODS

All amounts per 100g/100ml unless otherwise stated	Cal kcal	Pro g	Carb g	Fat g	Fibre g
SOFT DRINKS					
Apple & Blackcurrant Drink					
Quosh	**72**	Tr	16.6	Tr	n/a
Robinsons	**43.1**	Tr	9.7	Tr	n/a
no added sugar Robinsons	**8.5**	0.1	1.1	Tr	n/a
Banana For Milk Robinsons	**157.6**	Tr	38.9	Tr	n/a
no added sugar	**8.5**	0.1	1.3	Tr	n/a
Banana Nesquik, as sold Nestlé	**395**	0	97.3	0.5	0
fresh, each	**175**	8.1	26.7	3.9	0.7
Capri-Sun Juice Drink Capri-Sun					
apple	**46.8**	0	11.3	0	n/a
blackcurrant	**53**	0	12.9	0	n/a
orange	**44.8**	0	10.8	0	n/a
strawberry	**55.9**	0	13.6	0	n/a
tropical	**45.1**	Tr	10.9	0	n/a
wild berries	**46**	0	11.1	0	n/a
Chocolate Nesquik, as sold					
Nestlé	**377**	4.9	82.5	3	5
fresh, each	**190**	8.8	28.8	4.3	1.3
Crusha Silver Spoon					
banana	**127**	**0.7**	32	0.3	n/a
chocolate	**232**	**0.2**	47	0.7	n/a
lime	**126**	**0.7**	32	0.3	n/a
raspberry	**124**	**0.7**	31	0.3	n/a
strawberry	**127**	0.7	32	0.3	n/a

All amounts per 100g/100ml unless otherwise stated	Cal kcal	Pro g	Carb g	Fat g	Fibre g
Frijj Extreme Milkshakes,					
each DAIRY CREST					
chocolate	**70**	3.5	11.7	1	n/a
strawberry	**61**	3.4	10.1	0.8	n/a
Fruit Shoot ROBINSONS					
apple	**46.8**	Tr	11.3	Tr	n/a
apple, no added sugar	**6.4**	Tr	1.1	Tr	n/a
blackcurrant & apple	**56.7**	Tr	13.7	Tr	n/a
blackcurrant & apple,					
no added sugar	**4.9**	Tr	0.8	Tr	n/a
orange & peach	**50.4**	Tr	12.2	Tr	n/a
orange & peach, no added sugar	**5.2**	0.1	0.8	Tr	n/a
strawberry	**44.7**	Tr	10.6	n/a	n/a
strawberry, no added sugar	**5.2**	0.1	0.6	Tr	n/a
tropical, no added sugar	**6.4**	Tr	1	Tr	n/a
Splat Milkshakes, each AMBROSIA					
banana	**72**	2.6	12.6	1.2	0
milk chocolate	**80**	2.8	14.2	1.3	0.4
strawberry	**71**	2.6	12.5	1.2	0
Strawberry & Raspberry					
For Milk ROBINSONS	**137.2**	Tr	33.5	Tr	n/a
Strawberry Nesquik, as sold					
NESTLÉ	**390**	0	96.7	0.5	0
fresh, each	**175**	8.3	26	4	0.8

All amounts per 100g/100ml unless otherwise stated	Cal kcal	Pro g	Carb g	Fat g	Fibre g
Snoozoo Malted Food Drink,					
as sold GLAXO SMITHKLINE					
banana, caffeine free	**73**	2	15.1	0.9	0.5
chocolate	**74**	1.7	15	0.9	0.9
strawberry, caffeine free	**73**	2	15.3	0.9	0.5
Sunny Delight Drink,					
each PROCTER & GAMBLE					
Caribbean, no added sugar	**10**	Tr	1.6	0.2	Tr
Florida	**39**	Tr	8.9	0.1	Tr
Florida, no added sugar	**10**	Tr	1.4	0.2	Tr
Um Bongo Fruit Drink, each					
LIBBY	**43**	Tr	10.7	Tr	Tr

See also: **DRINKS (NON-ALCOHOLIC)**

DAIRY

Articlife Fromage Frais YOPLAIT	**93**	7.1	13.1	1.3	0.2
Articlife Whole Milk Yogurt					
YOPLAIT	**110**	3.7	17.5	2.8	n/a
Babybel, mini FROMAGERIES BEL	**299**	23	Tr	23	n/a
Cheestrings, all flavours					
GOLDEN VALE	**328**	28	Tr	24	n/a
Cheez Dippers FROMAGERIES BEL	**288**	11	25	16	n/a
Dairylea Cheese Rippers KRAFT	**260**	24.5	1.2	17	0

All amounts per 100g/100ml unless otherwise stated	Cal kcal	Pro g	Carb g	Fat g	Fibre g
Dairylea Cheese Strip Cheese KRAFT	**350**	21.5	1	27.5	0
Fromage Frais MÜLLER	**135**	6.1	13.5	6.3	n/a
Fruit Corner Snack Size, strawberry MÜLLER	**118**	3.7	17.1	3.9	n/a
Fruit Tumble, organic YEO VALLEY					
Apricot	**114**	5.1	13.3	4.5	0.2
Peach	**115**	5.2	13.3	4.5	0.2
Raspberry	**113**	5.1	13.1	4.5	0.4
Strawberry	**114**	5.1	13.2	4.5	0.2
Junior Yofu PROVAMEL					
Peach & Pear	**84**	3.8	12.4	2.2	1.2
Strawberry & Banana	**85**	3.8	12.7	2.2	1.2
Laughing Cow FROMAGERIES BEL	**269**	10	6.5	22.5	n/a
Light	**141**	13	6.5	7	n/a
Munch Bunch Fromage Frais NESTLÉ	**115**	7.7	14.3	2.9	0.2
Munch Bunch Wholemilk Yogurt NESTLÉ					
apricot	**108**	4.4	15.4	3.2	0.1
banana	**106**	4.3	15.1	3.1	0.4
blackcurrant	**107**	4.4	15.4	3.1	0.4
raspberry	**108**	4.4	15.5	3.2	0.1
strawberry	**108**	4.4	15.5	3.2	0.1

All amounts per 100g/100ml unless otherwise stated	Cal kcal	Pro g	Carb g	Fat g	Fibre g
Petits Filous Fromage Frais					
YOPLAIT	102	6.4	13	2.8	0.3
Layers	108	7.1	14	2.7	n/a
Petits Filous Frubes YOPLAIT	110	6.7	14	2.9	n/a
Pouches	94	3.2	14.8	2.4	n/a
Strawberry Jumble, organic					
YEO VALLEY					
Strawberry	114	5.1	13.2	4.5	0.2
Strawberry & Peach	115	5.2	13.3	4.5	0.2
Strawberry & Raspberry	114	5.1	13.2	4.5	0.3
Strawberry & Vanilla	114	5.2	13.2	4.5	0.2
Wildlife Fromage Frais	93	7.1	13.2	1.3	0.2
with Fruit Puree YOPLAIT	93	7.1	13.2	1.3	0.2
Winnie the Pooh Fromage Frais					
NESTLÉ	130	7.1	18.9	2.7	0.2
Winnie the Pooh Yogurt NESTLÉ					
apricot	109	4.3	16.1	3	0.1
raspberry	103	4.3	15.9	3	0.4
strawberry	109	4.3	16	3	0.1
Yop Yogurt Drink YOPLAIT					
Pineapple & Peach	79	2.8	14	1.3	n/a
Raspberry	79	2.8	14	1.3	n/a
Strawberry	79	2.8	14	1.3	n/a

See also: **DAIRY PRODUCTS**

All amounts per 100g/100ml unless otherwise stated	Cal kcal	Pro g	Carb g	Fat g	Fibre g

DESSERTS

Banana Nesquik Dessert,					
as sold NESTLÉ	**450**	3.7	74.6	15	0.3
Cadbury Buttons Twinpot MÜLLER	**280**	6.2	30.8	14.9	n/a
Fruitini Mixed Fruit Pieces					
DEL MONTE	**51**	0.4	12	0.1	n/a
in Juice	**51**	0.4	12	0.1	n/a
in Orange Jelly	**67**	0.1	15.8	0.1	n/a
in Strawberry Jelly	**65**	0.3	15.3	0.1	n/a
Fruit Express DEL MONTE					
mixed fruit in juice	**51**	0.4	12	0.1	n/a
peach & pear in juice	**47**	0.4	10.8	0.1	n/a
peach pieces in juice	**49**	0.5	11.5	0.1	n/a
pineapple chunks in light syrup	**65**	0.4	15	0.1	n/a
Jelly MÜLLER					
blackcurrant	**74**	0.9	17.7	Tr	n/a
orange	**76**	0.9	18	Tr	n/a
strawberry	**73**	0.9	17.4	Tr	n/a
Jelly Pots, ready to eat, each HARTLEY'S					
all flavours	**100**	0	25	0	n/a
low sugar, all flavours	**9**	0	2.3	0	n/a
Micro Donut Balls with Jam					
(frozen) MCCAIN	**358**	6	44.8	17.1	n/a
Micro Donut Rings & chocolate					
dip (frozen) MCCAIN	**337**	5.9	48.7	17.6	n/a

All amounts per 100g/100ml unless otherwise stated	Cal kcal	Pro g	Carb g	Fat g	Fibre g
Petits Filous Little Desserts					
YOPLAIT	**169**	4.7	23.6	6.3	n/a
Custard Dessert Pot AMBROSIA					
banana flavour	**102**	2.8	16.5	2.8	0
chocolate flavour	**114**	3.2	18.5	3	0
strawberry flavour	**102**	2.8	16.4	2.8	0
toffee flavour	**104**	2.8	16.8	2.8	0
vanilla flavour	**102**	2.8	16.4	2.8	0

ICE CREAM

Big Milk, each WALLS	**68**	3.3	21	7	0.6
Calippo, each WALLS					
Lime/Lemon	**54**	Tr	22.4	Tr	0.2
Orange	**89**	Tr	21.1	Tr	0.1
Strawberry	**93**	Tr	22.2	Tr	0.2
Fab, each NESTLÉ	**79**	0.3	13.2	2.7	n/a
Fruit Pastille Lolly, each NESTLÉ	**55**	0.1	13.4	Tr	Tr
Funny Foot, each WALLS	**83**	2	23	10	n/a
King Banana, each LYONS MAID	**140**	0.8	12	9.9	n/a
Lip Smacker, each LYONS MAID	**77**	0	19.4	0	n/a
Mickey, each LYONS MAID	**98**	2.2	11.7	4.7	n/a
Milkybar Ice Cream, each NESTLÉ	**114**	2	9.6	7.5	n/a

All amounts per 100g/100ml unless otherwise stated	Cal kcal	Pro g	Carb g	Fat g	Fibre g
Mini Milk, each WALLS					
chocolate	**29**	3.8	22.5	3	0.2
strawberry	**30**	3.8	22.5	4.1	0.4
vanilla	**30**	3.3	20.5	3.2	0.6
Mivi, each LYONS MAID					
pineapple & cream	**85**	1	13.8	2.8	n/a
raspberry & cream	**84**	1.2	13.5	2.8	n/a
strawberry & cream	**83**	1	13.4	2.7	n/a
Mr Men, each NESTLÉ					
milky strawberry	**55**	1.8	9	1.4	n/a
milky vanilla	**55**	1.8	8.9	1.3	n/a
orange	**30**	Tr	7.3	Tr	n/a
raspberry	**34**	Tr	8.4	0	n/a
Nobbly Bobbly, each LYONS MAID	**147**	1.4	22	5.9	n/a
Orange Maid, each LYONS MAID	**78**	0.3	19.1	0	n/a
Rocket, each WALLS	**40**	Tr	18.3	Tr	0.2
Sparkles, each WALLS	**50**	0	23	0	0.1
Twister, each WALLS	**77**	0	23	0	0.3
Zoom, each LYONS MAID	**46**	0.3	10	0.5	n/a

See also: **DESSERTS & PUDDINGS**

BISCUITS

Animals CADBURY	**495**	7	69.9	20.9	n/a

All amounts per 100g/100ml unless otherwise stated	Cal kcal	Pro g	Carb g	Fat g	Fibre g
Animal Bites CADBURY	**480**	7.1	69.8	19	n/a
BN Biscuit McVITIES					
chocolate	**460**	6	73	16	2.2
strawberry	**395**	5.8	78	6.8	1.3
vanilla	**470**	5.9	74	17	1.2
Chocolate Rings CADBURY	**510**	5.8	62.9	25.9	n/a
Happy Faces Biscuits,					
jam & cream JACOBS	**484**	4.8	66.1	22	1.6
Iced Gem JACOB'S	**388**	5	85.5	2.9	1.5
Jammie Dodger BURTON'S					
original	**437**	5.1	67.8	15.8	1.9
mini	**444**	6	73.5	14	1.7
vanilla thriller	**440**	5.2	68.1	16	1.8
vimto	**442**	5.4	68.4	16.3	1.7
Jam Rings CRAWFORD'S	**470**	5.5	73	17	1.9
Mallo's CADBURY	**465**	5.1	69.4	18.8	n/a
Party Rings FOX'S	**459**	5.1	75.8	15	n/a
Pink Wafers RIVINGTON	**534**	4.4	63.1	29.3	1.9
Wagon Wheels BURTON'S					
chocolate	**420**	5.4	67.3	14.8	2.2
jammie	**423**	5.2	67.8	14.3	2.1

See also: **BAKERY**

All amounts per 100g/100ml unless otherwise stated	Cal kcal	Pro g	Carb g	Fat g	Fibre g
SWEETS					
All Fruit Bars, each JORDANS					
apple & passionfruit	**88**	0.3	21.3	0.2	1.6
apple & strawberry	**89**	0.4	21.6	0.1	1.5
Bursting Bugs NESTLÉ	**333**	4.8	78.1	0.2	Tr
Buttons CADBURY	**525**	8	56	30	n/a
white	**555**	5	58	34	n/a
Dip Dab TREBOR BASSETT	**375**	0	90	0	n/a
Dolly Mixtures TREBOR BASSETT	**380**	2	86	3	n/a
Freddo CADBURY	**525**	8	56	30	n/a
Fruit Pastilles, Body Parts NESTLÉ	**368**	4.3	82.9	0	0
Hubba Bubba Chunks WRIGLEY					
Atomic Apple	**280**	0	n/a	0	0
Cool Cola	**295**	0	n/a	0	0
Serious Strawberry	**280**	0	n/a	0	0
Hubba Bubba Tapes WRIGLEY					
Cheeky Black Cherry	**300**	0	n/a	0	0
Snappy Strawberry	**290**	0	n/a	0	0
Jelly Babies	**334**	5.2	78	0	0
NESTLÉ	**356**	4.5	84.6	Tr	0
TREBOR BASSETT	**335**	4	80	0	n/a
Jellytots NESTLÉ	**346**	0.1	86.5	0	0
Milky Bar NESTLÉ	**542**	7.6	57.5	31.3	0

All amounts per 100g/100ml unless otherwise stated	Cal kcal	Pro g	Carb g	Fat g	Fibre g
Milky Way Magic Stars MARS	**522**	6.9	58.5	29	n/a
Quality Street NESTLÉ					
Big Green Triangle	**538**	7.2	55.4	31.9	1.1
Big Purple One	**489**	5	60.2	25.4	0.6
Big Toffee Finger	**471**	3	67.7	20.9	0.2
Smarties NESTLÉ	**458**	4.1	73.5	16.4	0.6
fruity	**398**	0.1	91.7	3.5	0
giant	**476**	4.6	70.4	19.6	0.7
Starburst Joosters MARS	**354**	0	89	0.1	0
Starburst Juicy Gums MARS	**309**	5.9	71	4.1	n/a
Taz CADBURY	**480**	4	61	25	n/a
Toffeepops BURTON'S	**461**	5	64.4	20.4	n/a
Winders, Real Fruit KELLOGG'S					
apple	**381**	0.3	77	8	2
blackcurrant	**381**	0.2	77	8	2
orange	**381**	0.3	77	8	2
raspberry	**379**	0.3	77	8	3
strawberry	**377**	0.3	76	8	2

See also: **SWEETS & CHOCOLATE**

TINNED PASTA

Pasta Shapes					
all varieties HP	**50**	1.5	10.6	0.2	0.2

All amounts per 100g/100ml unless otherwise stated	Cal kcal	Pro g	Carb g	Fat g	Fibre g
Funky Fish HP	**54**	1.4	11.6	0.3	0.4
Thomas the Tank Engine HEINZ	**53**	1.7	11	0.2	0.5
Tweenies HEINZ	**53**	1.7	11	0.2	0.5
Pasta shapes with sausages HEINZ					
Groovy Chick, in tomato sauce	**104**	3.2	12.7	4.5	0.5
Scoobie Doo, in tomato sauce	**99**	3.5	12.2	4	0.9
Space Spaghetti Shapes,					
in tomato sauce HP	**54**	1.4	11.6	0.3	0.4

See also: **PASTA**

POTATO PRODUCTS

Alphabites BIRDS EYE	**134**	2	19.5	5.3	1.4
Potato Smiles McCAIN	**225**	3.9	32	9	n/a

See also: **CHIPS, FRIES & SHAPED POTATO PRODUCTS**

DIPS

Dairylea Dunkers Breadstick, KRAFT	**235**	10.5	28	8.6	0.9
Dairylea Dunkers Jumbo Tubes KRAFT	**255**	9.2	26	12.5	0.8

See also: **DIPS & PRE-DRESSED SALADS**

All amounts per 100g/100ml unless otherwise stated	Cal kcal	Pro g	Carb g	Fat g	Fibre g
READY MEALS					
Bangers & Mash, bitesize, each					
BIRDS EYE	**294**	14	52	15	3
Captain's Coins Fish Burgers					
BIRDS EYE	**188**	9.5	18.7	8.3	1.1
Chicken Bites BIRDS EYE	**210**	18.6	5.8	12.5	0.2
Chicken Dippers BIRDS EYE	**219**	13.1	12	13.2	0.6
100% breast	**217**	13.7	13.5	12	0.4
Chicken Griddlers, original					
BIRDS EYE	**213**	15.7	4.8	14.5	0.2
BBQ	**209**	18.3	5.7	12.5	0.2
Chicken Korma & Rice, each					
BIRDS EYE	**310**	16	55	2.7	2.7
Chicken Nuggets	**281**	13	28	13	2
micro MCCAIN	**267**	16.7	19.8	14.2	n/a
Chicken O's BIRDS EYE	**231**	13	15.6	13	0.8
Chicksticks BIRDS EYE	**237**	13.9	16.7	12.7	0.8
Cod Fillet Fish Fingers BIRDS EYE	**186**	13	15.6	7.9	0.7
Crispy Pancakes FINDUS					
chicken, bacon & sweetcorn	**160**	5.5	26	4	1
minced beef	**160**	6.5	25	3.5	1
three cheeses	**190**	7	25	6.5	0.8

All amounts per 100g/100ml unless otherwise stated	Cal kcal	Pro g	Carb g	Fat g	Fibre g
Dairylea Lunchables each KRAFT					
chicken	**320**	19	19.5	18	0.8
ham	**325**	18.5	20	18	0.8
hotdog	**280**	12.5	18.5	17	0.6
Dinosaur Roll BERNARD MATTHEWS	**175**	11.1	9.8	10.2	0.3
Fish Fingers BIRDS EYE	**187**	12.7	16.7	7.7	0.7
YOUNG'S BLUECREST	**193**	10.7	17.7	8.8	0.8
Fishysaurus YOUNG'S BLUECREST	**201**	12.1	15.1	10.2	0.7
Flipper Dippers YOUNG'S BLUECREST	**229**	10	13.1	15.2	0.7
Flips FINDUS					
cheese & ham	**170**	6.5	25	4.5	n/a
chilli beef	**160**	7	23	4.5	n/a
Haddock Fillet Fish Fingers BIRDS EYE	**185**	12.5	15.6	8.1	0.7
Meatballs CAMPBELL'S					
in Awesome Onion Gravy	**83**	4.5	9.8	2.9	n/a
in Brilliant Bolognese Sauce	**93**	4.7	12.1	2.9	n/a
in Gorgeous Gravy	**82**	4.5	9.6	2.9	n/a
in Tasty Tomato Sauce	**91**	4.7	11.6	2.9	n/a
Princess Dreams BERNARD MATTHEWS	**175**	11.1	9.8	10.2	0.3
Salmon Fingers YOUNG'S BLUECREST	**199**	14.7	15.6	8.6	1.5
Shepherd's Pie, each BIRDS EYE	**230**	9.9	32	7.2	4.5
Soccer Slices BERNARD MATTHEWS	**175**	11.1	9.8	10.2	0.3

All amounts per 100g/100ml unless otherwise stated	Cal kcal	Pro g	Carb g	Fat g	Fibre g
Spaghetti Bolognese & Meatballs, each BIRDS EYE	**400**	14	52	15	3
Vegetable Fingers, Crispy BIRDS EYE	**191**	4.8	23.8	8.5	1.8
Wall's Balls WALL'S	**301**	13.8	21.3	17.8	0.8
cheese	**301**	13.8	21.3	17.8	0.8

See also: **SNACK MEALS, READY MEALS**

CRISPS/SNACKS

Cheesy Nibbles, per 10p pack	**77**	0.9	7.2	4.9	0.4
French Fries, per pack (22g) WALKERS					
Cheese & Onion	**94**	1.2	14.1	3.5	0.9
Ready Salted	**95**	1.1	14.1	3.7	1
Salt & Vinegar	**92**	1.1	13.9	3.5	1
Worcester Sauce	**92**	1.1	14.1	1.8	0.9
Hula Hoops, per pack (27g) all flavours UNITED BISCUITS	**175**	1.1	20.5	9.7	0.6
Krunchie Onion Rings, per 10p pack	**69**	0.9	8.4	3.5	0.4
Krunchie Sticks, per 10p pack	**66**	1.1	8.3	3.2	0.3
Monster Munch, per pack (25g) WALKERS					
Flamin' Hot	**123**	1.8	15	6.3	0.4
Pickled Onion	**124**	1.5	15.5	6.3	0.4
Roast Beef	**119**	1.7	14.5	6	0.4

All amounts per 100g/100ml unless otherwise stated	Cal kcal	Pro g	Carb g	Fat g	Fibre g
Oinks, per 10p pack	**70**	1.1	7.8	3.8	0.5
Petrified Prawns, per 10p pack	**70**	1	8.5	3.5	0.2
Potato Heads, per pack (23g) WALKERS					
Cheese & Onion	**105**	2.1	13	4.8	1.2
Prawn Cocktail	**104**	2	13	4.8	1.3
Ready Salted	**106**	2	13	4.8	1.4
Roast Chicken	**106**	2	13	4.8	0.4
Quarterbacks, per 10p pack	**72**	0.9	7.6	4.2	0.5
Skips, per pack (17g) UNITED BISCUITS					
Prawn Cocktail	**94**	0.6	10.9	5.4	0.3
Tangy Toms, per 10p pack	**70**	1	8.2	3.6	0.3
Transform A, per 10p pack					
Cheese & Onion	**73**	0.9	7.8	4.2	0.4
Pickled Onion	**69**	0.9	7.3	4	0.5
Spicy	**63**	1	8.6	2.7	0.3
Wotsits, per pack (21g) WALKERS					
Cheesy	**110**	1.7	11.3	6.3	0.2
Flamin' Hot	**109**	1.1	12	6.3	0.3
Mild Cheese (19g)	**102**	1.1	10.3	6.3	0.2
Prawn Cocktail (19g)	**99**	1	10.5	5.9	0.2
Twisted BBQ (22g)	**113**	1	12.5	6.6	0.3
Twisted Really Cheesy (22g)	**117**	1.3	12.1	7	0.2

FAMILY FAVOURITES & RECIPES

BEANBURGER, SOYA, FRIED IN VEGETABLE OIL

120g chopped onion	1 tsp mixed herbs
10g vegetable oil	20g soya sauce
320g boiled soya beans	35g tomato purée
75g porridge oats	1 egg
10g chopped fresh parsley	vegetable oil absorbed on frying (20g)

Fry onion in oil until brown. Mix beans and onions together
with remaining ingredients. Form into 6–8 shapes
approximately 1cm thick. Fry for 3 minutes either side.

Values per 100g: Cal 193, Pro 10.6, Carb 13.7, Fat 11.0, Fibre 4.7

BEEF BOURGUIGNONNE

1 tbsp vegetable oil	150g button mushrooms
100g button onions	5g tomato purée
1 clove garlic, crushed	1 tsp dried mixed herbs
500g stewing beef, diced	250ml red wine
50g streaky bacon rashers, chopped	250ml stock
15g flour	1/2 tsp salt
	1/4 tsp pepper

Brown the onions, garlic, meat and bacon in oil. Stir
in flour, tomato purée, mixed herbs, wine, stock and
seasoning. Bring to the boil, cover and simmer for 1 hour,
stirring occasionally. Add mushrooms and cook for a further
30 minutes.

Values per 100g: Cal 105, Pro 14.3, Carb 2.5, Fat 4.3, Fibre 0.4

BEEF STEW

500g stewing beef, diced	500ml stock
150g onions, chopped	150g carrots, chopped
1 tbsp vegetable oil	1/2 tsp salt
30g flour	1/4 tsp pepper

Brown the meat and onions in oil, add flour and cook for 1 minute. Blend in the stock, add carrots and seasoning, transfer to a dish, cover and cook in the oven for 2 hours at 180°C/mark 4.

Values per 100g: Cal 107, Pro 12.0, Carb 4.7, Fat 4.6, Fibre 0.7

BOLOGNESE SAUCE

1 clove garlic, crushed	397g canned tomatoes
60g onions, chopped finely	250ml stock
500g minced beef	2 tsp vegetable oil
40g carrots, chopped finely	1/2 tsp salt
30g celery, chopped finely	1/4 tsp pepper
10g tomato purée	1/4 tsp dried mixed herbs

Brown the garlic, onions and mince in oil, add carrots and celery. Stir in the other ingredients and simmer for 40 minutes with the lid on.

Values per 100g: Cal 161, Pro 11.8, Carb 2.5, Fat 11.6, Fibre 0.6

BREAD PUDDING

225g white bread
275ml milk
50g melted butter
75g demerara sugar

4g mixed spice
1 beaten egg
175g dried fruit

Break bread into pieces, cover with milk and leave for
30 minutes. Add remaining ingredients, mix well and bake
for 1¼ hours at 180°C/mark 4.

Values per 100g: Cal 289, Pro 5.9, Carb 48, Fat 9.5, Fibre 1.2

CAULIFLOWER CHEESE

100g grated cheese
1 small cauliflower (700g)
100ml cauliflower water
½ level tsp salt

25g margarine
25g flour
250ml semi-skimmed milk
pepper

Boil cauliflower until just tender, break into florets. Drain
saving 100ml water, place in a dish and keep warm. Make a
white sauce from the margarine, flour, milk and cauliflower
water. Add 75g cheese and season. Pour over the cauliflower
and sprinkle with the remaining cheese. Brown under a grill
or in a hot oven, 220°C/mark 7.

Values per 100g: Cal 102, Pro 6.0, Carb 5.1, Fat 6.5, Fibre 1.3

CASSEROLE, SAUSAGE

400g diced pork	227g baked beans,
150g onions, chopped	in tomato sauce, canned
200g streaky bacon rashers,	1 bay leaf
chopped	1 tsp dried mixed herbs
1 tbsp vegetable oil	300ml stock
200g pork sausage,	1/2 tsp salt
chopped	1/4 tsp pepper

Brown the pork, onions and bacon in the oil, add the remaining ingredients and bake, uncovered, for 1 1/2 hours at 170°C/mark 3.

Values per 100g: Cal 165, Pro 11.9, Carb 5.1, Fat 10.9, Fibre 0.9

CASSEROLE, VEGETABLE

240g diced potato	90g canned sweetcorn
120g sliced carrot	90g frozen peas
120g diced onion	90g chopped tomatoes
120g diced swede	450g canned tomatoes
120g diced parsnip	1 tsp marmite

Place all ingredients in a casserole and stir. Cover and cook for approximately 1 hour at 190°C/mark 5.

Values per 100g: Cal 52, Pro 2.2, Carb 10.6, Fat 0.4, Fibre 2.1

CHILLI CON CARNE

500g minced beef	15ml vinegar
150g onions, chopped	1 tsp sugar
100g green peppers, chopped	30g tomato purée
1 tbsp vegetable oil	397g canned tomatoes
1 tsp salt	150ml stock
¼ tsp pepper	115g red kidney beans, canned, drained

Brown the mince, onions and peppers in oil. Blend the other ingredients and stir into the meat. Cover and simmer gently for 40 minutes. Add the kidney beans and continue cooking for a further 10 minutes.

Values per 100g: Cal 121, Pro 9.2, Carb 4.4, Fat 7.5, Fibre 1.1

COQ AU VIN

100g back bacon rashers, chopped	½ tsp salt
1000g chicken leg quarters (weighed with bone)	¼ tsp pepper
50g butter	100g shallots
50g flour	1 tsp dried mixed herbs
	100g button mushrooms
	600ml red wine

Brown the bacon and chicken coated in seasonal flour, in butter. Add the shallots, mixed herbs and red wine, cover and simmer for 35–45 minutes. Add the mushrooms and cook for another 20 minutes.

Values per 100g: Cal 155, Pro 11.1, Carb 3.2, Fat 11, Fibre 0.3

CRUMBLE, FRUIT, PLAIN OR WHOLEMEAL

400g prepared fruit	100g plain or wholemeal flour
50g margarine	100g sugar

Prepare fruit. Arrange in a dish and sprinkle with sugar.
Rub together the other ingredients and pile on top. Bake for
40 minutes at 190°C/mark 5.

Values per 100g: Cal 195, Pro 2.6, Carb 31.6, Fat 7.4, Fibre 2.7

CURRY, BEEF

1 clove garlic, crushed	½ tsp ground cumin
60g onions, chopped	½ tsp ground turmeric
500g lean braising steak, diced	8g root ginger, ground
	300ml water
1 tbsp vegetable oil	½ tsp salt
1 tbsp ground coriander	5ml lemon juice
1 tsp chilli powder	1 tsp garam masala

Brown the garlic, onions and meat in oil. Add spices and
ginger. Stir in water, salt and lemon juice, cover and bring to
the boil. Cook for 1½ hours stirring occasionally. Add garam
masala.

Values per 100g: Cal 143, Pro 18.8, Carb 1, Fat 7.1, Fibre 0.2

CURRY, CHICK PEA DAHL

225g dry chick pea dahl	1 tsp chilli powder
220ml water absorbed	1/2 tsp garam masala
on soaking	7g chopped green chilli
28g vegetable oil	100g chopped tomato
60g chopped onion	415ml water
2g crushed garlic	

Soak the chick pea dahl overnight. Fry the onion and garlic until brown. Add a little water together with spices and tomatoes. Stir and cook until dry. Add dahl and water, simmer until cooked.

Values per 100g: Cal 154, Pro 7.9, Carb 17.9, Fat 6.1, Fibre N

CURRY, LAMB, MADE WITH CANNED CURRY SAUCE

500g stewing lamb, diced	385g curry sauce, canned
1 tbsp vegetable oil	

Brown the lamb in oil. Add the sauce, cover and simmer for 45 minutes.

Values per 100g: Cal 249, Pro 11, Carb 3.6, Fat 13.4, Fibre N

FISH PIE

200g cooked cod	Sauce:
400g mashed potato	150ml milk
	15g margarine
	15g flour
	½ level tsp salt

Flake the fish and mix with the white sauce. Pipe a potato border round a dish, pour in the fish mixture. Brown in the oven, 200°C/mark 6, for 30 minutes.

Values per 100g: Cal 102, Pro 8, Carb 12.3, Fat 3.0, Fibre 0.7

FRENCH DRESSING

25ml vinegar	½ level tsp salt
75g olive oil	½ level tsp pepper

Shake the ingredients together in a screw-topped jar or bottle.

Values per 100g: Cal 462, Pro 0.1, Carb 4.5, Fat 49.4, Fibre 0

FRUIT CAKE, RICH

200g margarine	250g flour
200g brown sugar	¼ tsp salt
4 eggs	750g mixed fruit
20g black treacle	150g mixed glacé fruit,
20ml brandy	chopped
1 tsp mixed spice	

Cream the fat and sugar. Beat the eggs, treacle and brandy. Fold in the sifted flour and spices and mix in the fruit. Turn into a 20cm cake tin. Bake for 4 hours at 150°C/mark 2.

Values per 100g: Cal 343, Pro 3.9, Carb 59.9, Fat 11.4, Fibre 1.5

FRUIT PIE, PASTRY TOP AND BOTTOM

450g raw shortcrust pastry	450g fruit (eg. apple, gooseberry, rhubarb, plum)
80g sugar	

Line a pie dish with half the pastry. Fill with prepared fruit and sugar and cover with remaining pastry. Bake for 10–15 minutes at 220°C/mark 7 to set pastry, then for about 20–30 minutes at 180°C/mark 4 to cook the fruit.

Values per 100g: Cal 260, Pro 3, Carb 34, Fat 13, Fibre 1.8

FRUIT SALAD

400g eating apples	200g bananas
113g grapes	120g kiwi fruit
320g oranges	113g strawberries
40ml lemon juice	

Syrup

57g caster sugar	114ml water

Dissolve the sugar in the water in a pan over a low heat. Bring to the boil and simmer for a minute, then remove from the heat and allow to cool. Prepare fruit and sprinkle with lemon juice. Mix fruit with the cool syrup and refrigerate.

Values per 100g: Cal 60, Pro 0.7, Carb 14.8, Fat 0.1, Fibre 1.3

GARLIC MUSHROOMS

250g mushrooms
2g garlic
40g butter

Clean mushrooms and remove stems. Crush the garlic and sauté in butter. Fill mushroom caps with the garlic butter mixture and grill for 5–7 minutes.

Values per 100g: Cal 140, Pro 2.1, Carb 0.7, Fat 14.4, Fibre 1.2

IRISH STEW

500g lamb neck fillet, diced	1 tsp dried mixed herbs
150g onions, sliced	15g flour
200g carrots, sliced	1/2 tsp salt
500g potatoes, sliced	1/4 tsp pepper
1 tbsp fresh parsley, chopped	300ml stock

Make layers of meat, vegetables, herbs, flour and seasoning in a casserole dish, ending with a top layer of potatoes. Pour in stock and cover. Bake for 1 hour at 170°C/mark 3, remove lid and cook for a further 30 minutes.

Values per 100g: Cal 107, Pro 7.7, Carb 8.6, Fat 4.9, Fibre 1

KEDGEREE

200g smoked haddock, cooked	2 eggs
100g boiled white rice	25g margarine
	1/2 tsp salt

Hard boil one egg. Melt the margarine and stir in the haddock, rice, salt and one beaten egg. Stir in chopped hard boiled egg and heat thoroughly.

Values per 100g: Cal 176, Pro 16, Carb 8, Fat 9.1, Fibre 0

LANCASHIRE HOTPOT

500g stewing lamb, diced	100g onions, sliced
1/2 tsp salt	500g potatoes, sliced
1/4 tsp pepper	300ml stock
100g carrots, sliced	2 tsp vegetable oil
100g turnip, chopped	

Season the meat and mix with carrots, turnip and onions. Layer this with the potatoes in a casserole, beginning and ending with potatoes. Add stock and brush the top with oil. Cover and bake for 2 hours at 150°C/mark 2. Remove lid to brown the potatoes for the last 30 minutes.

Values per 100g: Cal 119, Pro 7.4, Carb 7.4, Fat 6.9, Fibre 0.9

LASAGNE

Meat sauce:
1 tbsp vegetable oil
50g streaky bacon rashers, chopped
50g onions, chopped
50g carrots, chopped
30g celery, chopped
300g minced beef
220g canned tomatoes
375ml stock
1 clove garlic, crushed
1/2 tsp salt
1/4 tsp pepper
1/2 tsp marjoram
1 bay leaf
50g mushrooms, sliced

Cheese sauce:
30g margarine
30g flour
400ml milk
75g cheese, grated

200g lasagne, raw

To top:
25g cheese, grated

Brown the bacon, onions, carrots, celery and mince in the oil. Stir in the remaining ingredients for the meat sauce and simmer for 15 minutes. For the cheese sauce, melt the margarine, add flour and cook for a few minutes, stir in the milk and cheese and cook gently until mixture thickens. In a dish, add alternative layers of lasagne, meat and cheese sauce ending with a layer of lasagne and cheese sauce. Sprinkle with cheese and bake for 1 hour at 190°C/mark 5.

Values per 100g: Cal 191, Pro 9.8, Carb 14.6, Fat 10.8, Fibre 0.8

MACARONI CHEESE

280g cooked macaroni	25g flour
350ml milk	100g grated cheese
25g margarine	½ tsp salt

Boil the macaroni and drain well. Make a white sauce from the margarine, flour and milk. Add 75g of the cheese and season. Add the macaroni and put in a pie dish. Sprinkle with remaining cheese and brown under grill or in a hot oven at 220°C/mark 7.

Values per 100g: Cal 162, Pro 6.7, Carb 12.2, Fat 9.9, Fibre 0.5

MILK PUDDING (RICE, SAGO, SEMOLINA OR TAPIOCA)

500ml whole milk	50g rice, sago, semolina
25g sugar	or tapioca

Simmer until cooked or bake in a moderate oven at 180°C/mark 4.

Values per 100g: Cal 130, Pro 4.1, Carb 19.6, Fat 4.3, Fibre 0.1

NUT ROAST

90g chopped onion	225g chopped mixed nuts
11g vegetable oil	115g wholemeal
20g flour	breadcrumbs
140ml water	1 tsp marmite
	1 tsp mixed herbs

Fry onion in the oil. Add flour and water and thicken. Mix in nuts, breadcrumbs, marmite and herbs. Pack into a loaf tin and cover with foil. Bake at 190°C/mark 5 for 35–45 minutes.

Values per 100g: Cal 333, Pro 13.2, Carb 18.4, Fat 23.5, Fibre 4.1

OMELETTE

2 eggs	½ tsp salt
10ml water	pepper
10g butter	

Beat eggs with salt and water. Heat butter in an omelette pan. Pour in the mixture and stir until it begins to thicken evenly. While still creamy, fold the omelette and serve.

Values per 100g: Cal 195, Pro 10.9, Carb Tr, Fat 16.8, Fibre 0

OMELETTE, CHEESE

115g omelette, cooked
60g Cheddar cheese

Proportions are derived from recipe review.

Values per 100g: Cal 271, Pro 15.9, Carb Tr, Fat 23, Fibre 0

PANCAKES, SAVOURY

112g flour   56g lard (for pan)
300ml whole milk   ¼ tsp salt
1 egg

Method as for sweet pancakes.

Values per 100g: Cal 255, Pro 6.4, Carb 23.9, Fat 15.5, Fibre 0.8

PANCAKES, SWEET

100g flour   50g lard (for pan)
250ml whole milk   50g sugar
1 egg

Sieve the flour into a basin, add the egg and about 100ml of
the milk, stirring until smooth. Add the rest of the milk and
beat to a smooth batter. Heat a little of the lard in a frying pan
and pour in enough batter to cover the bottom. Cook both
sides and turn onto sugared paper. Dredge lightly with sugar.
Repeat until all the batter is used, to give about 10 pancakes.

Values per 100g: Cal 302, Pro 6, Carb 34.9, Fat 16.3, Fibre 0.8

PASTRY, SHORTCRUST

200g flour	½ tsp salt
50g margarine	30ml water
50g lard	

Rub the fat into the flour, mix to a stiff dough with the water, roll out and bake at 200°C/mark 6.

Values per 100g: Cal 524, Pro 6.6, Carb 54.3, Fat 32.6, Fibre 2.2

PIZZA, CHEESE AND TOMATO

Dough:

200g flour
1 tsp salt
1 tsp sugar
150ml warm water
15g fresh yeast or
 2 tsp dried yeast

Topping:

200g tomatoes
150g cheese
8 black olives (40g)
20g oil

Make the dough, proving once. Knead and roll out shape. Leave for 10 minutes. Arrange sliced or pulped tomatoes on top, then cheese and olives. Brush with oil. Bake for 30 minutes at 230°C/mark 8.

Values per 100g: Cal 234, Pro 9.4, Carb 24.8, Fat 11.5, Fibre n/a

QUICHE, Cheese and Egg, Plain or Wholemeal

200g raw plain or wholemeal 150g milk
  shortcrust pastry 3 eggs
150g cheese

Line a 20cm flan ring with the shortcrust pastry. Fill with
grated cheese. Beat eggs in the warmed milk and pour into
pastry case. Bake for 10 minutes at 200°C/mark 6 and then
30 minutes at 180°C/mark 4.

Values per 100g: Cal 315, Pro 12.4, Carb 17.1, Fat 22.3, Fibre 0.6

QUICHE LORRAINE

200g raw shortcrust pastry 100g streaky bacon
2 eggs 100g cheese
200ml milk

Line a 20cm flan ring with shortcrust pastry. Fill with the fried,
chopped bacon and grated cheese. Beat the eggs in warmed
milk and pour into the pastry case. Bake for 10 minutes at
200°C/mark 6, then for 30 minutes at 180°C/mark 4.

Values per 100g: Cal 358, Pro 13.7, Carb 19.6, Fat 25.5, Fibre 0.7

RICE, EGG FRIED

35g vegetable oil   1½ beaten eggs
45g chopped onion   350g cooked white rice

Heat oil, add egg and remaining ingredients. Cook, turning mixture over, for 3 minutes.

Values per 100g: Cal 208, Pro 4.2, Carb 25.7, Fat 10.6, Fibre 0.4

RICE, FRIED WHITE

550g boiled rice   2g salt
168g chopped onion   ¼ tsp pepper
2 tbsp vegetable oil   1g spices
21g garlic

Fry onion and garlic until soft. Add boiled rice and seasoning. Fry until oil has been absorbed and rice is fully coated.

Values per 100g: Cal 144, Pro 2.5, Carb 25.9, Fat 4.1, Fibre 0.5

RICE PUDDING see **MILK PUDDING**

SALAD, GREEN

150g shredded lettuce   160g sliced green pepper
230g sliced cucumber   30g sliced celery

Toss all ingredients together.

Values per 100g: Cal 12, Pro 0.7, Carb 1.8, Fat 0.3, Fibre 1.0

SAGO PUDDING see MILK PUDDING

SAUCE, CHEESE

350ml whole or semi-skimmed milk	25g flour
75g cheese	25g margarine
1/2 level tsp salt	cayenne pepper

Melt the fat in a pan, add flour and cook gently for a few minutes stirring all the time. Add milk and cook until mixture thickens, stirring continually. Add grated cheese and seasoning. Reheat to soften the cheese, serve immediately.

Values per 100ml:

(whole milk) Cal 198, Pro 8.1, Carb 8.7, Fat 14.8, Fibre 0.2
(semi-skimmed) Cal 181, Pro 8.2, Carb 8.8, Fat 12.8, Fibre 0.2

SAUCE, WHITE SAVOURY

350ml whole or semi-skimmed milk	1/2 level tsp salt
25g flour	25g margarine

Melt fat in a pan. Add flour and cook for a few minutes stirring constantly. Add milk and salt, and cook gently until mixture thickens.

Values per 100ml:

(whole milk) Cal 151, Pro 4.2, Carb 10.6, Fat 10.3, Fibre 0.2
(semi-skimmed) Cal 130, Pro 4.4, Carb 10.7, Fat 8, Fibre 0.2

SAUCE, White Sweet

350ml whole or semi-
  skimmed milk
25g flour

25g margarine
30g sugar

As savoury white sauce except adding sugar and omitting salt.

Values per 100ml:

(whole milk) Cal 171, Pro 3.9, Carb 18.3, Fat 9.5, Fibre 0.2
(semi-skimmed) Cal 152, Pro 4, Carb 18.5, Fat 7.4, Fibre 0.2

SCONES, Plain

200g flour
4 tsp baking powder
¼ tsp salt

50g margarine
10g sugar
125ml milk

Sift the flour, sugar and baking powder and rub in fat. Mix in the milk. Roll out and cut into rounds. Bake in a hot oven at 220°C/mark 7 for about 10 minutes.

Values per 100g: Cal 364, Pro 7.2, Carb 53.7, Fat 14.8, Fibre 1.8

SCRAMBLED EGGS WITH MILK

2 eggs
15ml milk

20g butter
½ level tsp salt

Melt butter in pan, stir in beaten egg, milk and seasoning. Cook over gentle heat until mixture thickens.

Values per 100g: Cal 257, Pro 10.9, Carb 0.7, Fat 23.4, Fibre 0

SEMOLINA PUDDING see **MILK PUDDING**

SHEPHERD'S PIE

350g cooked minced beef	150ml water
100g onion boiled and chopped	50ml milk
	20g margarine
500g boiled potatoes	2 level tsp salt; pepper

Mix the beef and onion, moisten with water and add seasoning. Place in a pie dish. Mash the potato with the milk and margarine. Pile on top of the meat and bake in the oven for 25 minutes to brown, 190°C/mark 5.

Values per 100g: Cal 118, Pro 8, Carb 8.2, Fat 6.2, Fibre 0.6

SHORTBREAD

200g flour	100g butter
50g caster sugar	

Beat the butter and sugar to a cream. Mix in the flour and knead until smooth. Press into a flat tin to about 2cms thick. Bake for about 45 minutes at 170°C/mark 3.

Values per 100g: Cal 498, Pro 5.9, Carb 63.9, Fat 26.1, Fibre 1.9

SPONGE CAKE

150g flour	150g caster sugar
1 tsp baking powder	3 eggs
150g margarine	

Cream the fat and sugar until light and fluffy. Add the beaten egg a little at a time and beat well. Fold in the sifted flour and baking powder. Bake for about 20 minutes at 190°C/mark 5.

Values per 100g: Cal 467, Pro 6.3, Carb 52.4, Fat 27.2, Fibre 0.9

TAPIOCA PUDDING see MILK PUDDING

VEGETABLE PIE

100g chopped onion	200g canned tomatoes
100g sliced carrot	100ml water
100g sliced courgettes	2 tsp cornflour
60g chopped celery	1 tsp mixed herbs
50g sliced mushrooms	1 tsp marmite
80g chopped red pepper	300g raw shortcrust pastry
100g potatoes	

Place vegetables in a pan, together with herbs and marmite. Bring to the boil and simmer for 20–25 minutes. Make cornflour into a paste, add to pan, boil and stir until mixture thickens. Pour into pie dish and leave to cool. Roll pastry to fit dish size. Cut an additional 1 inch strip from remaining pastry, wet and place around the edge of the dish. Cover with pastry top and seal edges. Bake at 200°C/mark 6 for 30–40 minutes.

Values per 100g: Cal 159, Pro 3, Carb 18.8, Fat 8.4, Fibre 1.5

INDEX